O R M

OXFORD RESPIRATORY MEDICINE LIBRARY

O R M L

OXFORD RESPIRATORY MEDICINE LIBRARY

A Practical Guide to the Interpretation of Cardiopulmonary Exercise Tests

William Kinnear

Consultant Respiratory Physician, Queens Medical Centre,
Nottingham University Hospitals NHS Trust

John Blakey

Senior Lecturer, Liverpool School of Tropical Medicine
Honorary Consultant Respiratory Physician,
Aintree University Hospitals NHS Trust

OXFORD
UNIVERSITY PRESS

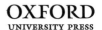

OXFORD
UNIVERSITY PRESS

Great Clarendon Street, Oxford, OX2 6DP,
United Kingdom

Oxford University Press is a department of the University of Oxford.
It furthers the University's objective of excellence in research, scholarship,
and education by publishing worldwide. Oxford is a registered trade mark of
Oxford University Press in the UK and in certain other countries

Published in the United States of America by Oxford University Press
198 Madison Avenue, New York, NY 10016, United States of America

British Library Cataloguing in Publication Data

Data available

Library of Congress Control Number: 2013957513

ISBN 978–0–19–870246–7

Printed in Great Britain by
Clays Ltd, St Ives plc

Contents

Preface

People are usually breathless when they are doing something, so it makes more sense to make measurements during exercise rather than relying on investigations performed at rest. Cardiopulmonary exercise testing is therefore an excellent way to work out why someone is breathless and to quantify their limitation.

Maximum oxygen uptake during exercise is also one of the best predictors of operative mortality and of prognosis in chronic cardiac or respiratory disease (as well as being an excellent measure of overall fitness in athletes). The cardiopulmonary exercise test (CPEX), during which VO_2max is routinely measured, is an increasingly common component of preoperative assessment and the management of patients with chronic lung or heart problems.

This book is a guide for clinicians and works logically through the main parameters that are measured during a CPEX. The physiology behind the calculation of these parameters is explained, so that interpretation of the results is based on a full understanding of the scientific principles from which they are derived. Clinical scenarios, key points, and practical tips all make this book easy to follow.

The first section of the book discusses the indications for a CPEX, the phases of the test, and how it should be supervised.

The second section analyses ten key CPEX parameters: five primary measurements (oxygen uptake, heart rate, ventilation, carbon dioxide output, and peripheral oxygen saturation (SpO_2)), three derived indices (oxygen (O_2) pulse, the respiratory exchange ratio, and ventilatory equivalents), and two thresholds (the anaerobic threshold and the respiratory compensation point).

The third section discusses how to integrate the results of a CPEX into a clinical report to help the referring clinician, with advice on the prescription of exercise.

Little prior knowledge of the subject is assumed, but by the end of the book, the reader will know what is going on in each of the plots of a standard nine-panel CPEX display. They will be able to look at this display and decide what is limiting exercise.

Glossary

Acidaemia—the fall in pH (or rise in hydrogen ion concentration) of the blood, as seen towards the end of a cardiopulmonary exercise test when the production of carbon dioxide and the generation of lactic acid exceed the buffering capacity of the body.

Anaerobic threshold (AT)—the point during a cardiopulmonary exercise test beyond which the oxygen demand of the muscles exceeds the amount delivered to them, so that they start to supplement aerobic with anaerobic metabolism.

Carbon dioxide output (VCO_2)—the volume of carbon dioxide (ml/min) exhaled through the lungs.

Heart rate reserve (HR reserve)—the difference between the predicted and observed maximum heart rate during a cardiopulmonary exercise test.

Maximum oxygen uptake (VO_2max)—the highest value of oxygen uptake (see below) seen during a cardiopulmonary exercise test.

Oxygen pulse (O_2 pulse)—oxygen uptake (see below) divided by heart rate, giving the amount of oxygen taken up from the lungs into the blood with each heart beat (ml/beat).

Oxygen uptake (VO_2)—the volume of oxygen (ml/min) taken up from the lungs into the blood.

Respiratory compensation point (RCP)—the point beyond which there is respiratory compensation for metabolic acidaemia, with a reduction in pH (or rise in hydrogen ion concentration), stimulating ventilation.

Respiratory exchange ratio (RER)—the ratio of carbon dioxide output to oxygen uptake.

Ventilation (VE)—minute ventilation (l/min).

Ventilatory equivalents (VEq)—the number of millilitres of ventilation required to get one millilitre of oxygen into (or carbon dioxide out of) the body.

Ventilatory reserve—the difference between the predicted and observed maximum minute ventilation during a cardiopulmonary exercise test.

Workload—the external work (joules/s or watts) done against the resistance of the cycle ergometer.

Abbreviations

ACSM	American College of Sports Medicine
AT	anaerobic threshold
H_2O	water
HCO_3^-	bicarbonate
bpm	beats per minute
CaO_2	oxygen content of arterial blood
CO_2	carbon dioxide
COPD	chronic obstructive pulmonary disease
CPEX	cardiopulmonary exercise test
CvO_2	oxygen content of mixed venous blood
ECG	electrocardiogram
FEV1	forced expiratory volume in one second
H^+	hydrogen ion(s)
Hb	haemoglobin
HCM	hypertrophic cardiomyopathy
HDL	high-density lipoprotein
HR	heart rate
kg	kilogram
kPa	kilopascal
l	litre
LDL	low-density lipoprotein
MET	metabolic equivalent; expressing work done as a multiple of resting energy expenditure
min	minute
ml	millilitre
O_2	oxygen
$PaCO_2$	arterial carbon dioxide partial pressure
PaO_2	arterial oxygen partial pressure
PO_2	oxygen partial pressure
PvO_2	mixed venous oxygen partial pressure
Q	lung perfusion
RCP	respiratory compensation point
RER	respiratory exchange ratio

s	second
SpO_2	peripheral oxygen saturation
V	ventilation
VCO_2	carbon dioxide output
Vd	dead space volume
VE	minute ventilation
VEmax	maximum minute ventilation
VEq	ventilatory equivalents
$VEqCO_2$	ventilatory equivalents for CO_2
$VEqO_2$	ventilatory equivalents for O_2
VO_2	oxygen uptake
VO_2max	maximum oxygen uptake
Vt	tidal volume
W	watt
yr	year

Part 1

Introduction

Chapter 1

Why do a cardiopulmonary exercise test?

> **Key points**
> - A cardiopulmonary exercise test (CPEX) involves measurements of cardiac and respiratory function whilst the subject exercises up to their maximum capacity.
> - A CPEX can be a useful tool for diagnosing heart and lung disease, working out why someone is breathless, and quantifying fitness.
> - Preoperative CPEX testing allows stratification of surgical risk and planning of post-operative care.

1.1 What is a CPEX?

In a cardiac exercise test, a patient with known or suspected coronary artery disease runs on a treadmill whilst their electrocardiogram (ECG) is monitored for ST segment changes. 'Cardiopulmonary' exercise tests (CPEX) go a step further by attaching a mask (or mouthpiece) to record breathing. This gives lots more information, not just about the lungs and heart, but also about the brain, peripheral circulation, leg muscles, etc. Clearly, if changes develop on the ECG during a CPEX, this is a strong pointer to the presence of heart disease; but these changes will not be discussed in any great detail in this book.

1.2 Key measurements

A CPEX can generate many numbers and graphs, but most of the useful information is derived from the five measurements described in Box 1.1.

> **Box 1.1 Key CPEX measurements**
> 1. The volume of air breathed in and out (minute ventilation (VE))
> 2. The volume of oxygen used up by the body (oxygen uptake; VO_2)
> 3. The volume of carbon dioxide produced (VCO_2)
> 4. Heart rate (HR)
> 5. Oxygen saturation (SpO_2).

Three more indices can be derived by combining two of these five measurements (the respiratory exchange ratio, oxygen (O_2) pulse and ventilatory equivalents). These eight parameters are also used to obtain a couple of useful thresholds (the anaerobic threshold (AT) and respiratory compensation point (RCP)). So CPEX interpretation, at an introductory level, requires an understanding of only ten parameters.

1.3 Why do a CPEX?

Most patients with cardiac or respiratory problems have symptoms which are worse on exertion, whereas many diagnostic tests are done when they are sitting in a chair or lying on a couch. It makes much more sense to make some measurements when they are exercising. A CPEX also puts the cardiac and respiratory systems under stress, so that the reserve capacity of the body can be assessed, particularly in terms of its ability to deliver oxygen to peripheral tissues (Box 1.2).

Box 1.2 Reasons for doing a CPEX

CPEX is a useful tool for:
1. Finding out what is wrong with patients who are short of breath
2. Assessing the contribution of cardiac or respiratory pathologies to incapacity
3. Quantifying the extent of the impairment
4. Assessing the risk to the patients of a surgical procedure
5. Measuring the response to an intervention.

As more and more exercise tests are performed, a wider range of clinicians need to develop some expertise in looking at the results. CPEX results can be a bit daunting. In this book, the different parameters are considered in detail, looking at the underlying physiology as needed, to see how they enable conclusions to be drawn about the patient's performance (Box 1.3 and Box 1.4).

Box 1.3 CPEX pointers to the presence of heart disease

- Reduced exercise capacity
  (low maximum VO_2 (VO_2max)—Chapter 3)
- HR rises rapidly
  (no HR reserve at peak exercise—Chapter 4)
- Impaired ventricular stroke volume
  (minimal rise in O_2 pulse—Chapter 5)
- Low cardiac output, with poor delivery of O_2 to muscle
  (anaerobic threshold occurs early—Chapter 9)
- Exercise not limited by breathing
  (VE doesn't reach predicted level—Chapter 6)
- Inefficient ventilation, with high ratio of dead space volume (Vd) to tidal volume (Vt)
  (high ventilatory equivalents—Chapter 10)

Box 1.4 CPEX pointers to the presence of lung disease
• Reduced exercise capacity   (low VO_2max—Chapter 3)   • Exercise not limited by cardiac output   (HR doesn't reach predicted—Chapter 4)   • Exercise limited by breathing   (no reserve in VE at peak exercise—Chapter 6)   • Exercise often stops as soon as muscles become anaerobic   (VE cannot increase in response to CO_2 production—Chapter 9)   • Inefficient ventilation, with high ratio of Vd to Vt   (high ventilatory equivalents—Chapter 10)   • Limited rise in Vt   (Chapter 6)   • Impaired ability to increase ventilation in response to acidaemia   (no RCP—Chapter 11)   • Desaturation   (Chapter 12)

1.4 Things that are not covered in this book

1.4.1 **Invasive measurements**

Measurements that involve insertion of central venous catheters, arterial lines, or blood sampling are beyond the scope of this volume. Similarly, tests where the subject inhales supplementary O_2—or indeed air with an artificially low O_2 content—are much more complicated to interpret and are beyond the scope of this introductory textbook.

1.4.2 **Technical aspects**

The technical aspects of a CPEX (how the analysers work, calibration, setting up the equipment, working out the ramp rate and so on) will not be discussed in any detail. This book is mainly about how to interpret the results.

1.4.3 **Shuttle and corridor walks, etc.**

This book focuses on the various measurements made during a full CPEX. Other ways of assessing exercise capacity—such as corridor or shuttle walks—will not be discussed, although clearly the physiological principles are equally applicable to the interpretation of these simpler tests.

1.5 Things to do first

Prior to a diagnostic CPEX, a detailed history and meticulous clinical examination are mandatory. A few basic tests (such as a chest X-ray, ECG, haemoglobin (Hb) concentration, and renal function), will have been performed, with arterial blood gases if there is any clinical suspicion of respiratory failure or a low resting SpO_2.

Whilst most patients will have spirometry and a flow-volume loop prior to a CPEX, whether more detailed tests will be performed will depend upon local practice and on the clinical indication for the test. Usually, static lung volumes and the carbon monoxide transfer factor will be measured first, with an ECG or other cardiac investigation if there is any clinical suspicion of heart failure.

These preliminaries are important. Whilst it may be possible to infer from CPEX results that the patient might be anaemic, have renal failure, intermittent claudication, or a muscle disease, there are other (better) ways of working this out.

Practical tip

A careful clinical assessment and a few simple tests beforehand will make interpretation of a CPEX very much easier.

Further reading

Abidov A, Rozanski A, Hachamovitch R, Hayes SW, Aboul-Enein F, Cohen I, et al. Prognostic significance of dyspnea in patients referred for cardiac stress testing. N Engl J Med. 2005 Nov 3;353(18):1889–98. PubMed PMID: 16267320.

Albouaini K, Egred M, Alahmar A, Wright DJ. Cardiopulmonary exercise testing and its application. Heart. 2007 Oct;93(10):1285–92. PubMed PMID: 17890705.

ERS Task Force, Palange P, Ward SA, Carlsen KH, Casaburi R, Gallagher CG, et al. Recommendations on the use of exercise testing in clinical practice. Eur Respir J. 2007 Jan;29(1):185–209. PubMed PMID: 17197484.

Parshall MB, Schwartzstein RM, Adams L, Banzett RB, Manning HL, Bourbeau J, et al. An official American Thoracic Society statement: update on the mechanisms, assessment, and management of dyspnea. Am J Respir Crit Care Med. 2012 Feb 15;185(4):435–52. PubMed PMID: 22336677.

Chapter 2

How to do a cardiopulmonary exercise test

Key points

Features of a standard cardiopulmonary exercise test (CPEX) are:
- cycle ergometer
- incremental ramp increase in load
- continue to maximum effort
- limited by symptoms
- results presented in a breath-by-breath format.

2.1 Cycle ergometers and treadmills

Over the years, many different exercise protocols and measurement techniques have been used. This variation hasn't made the topic easier to understand. These days, most CPEX tests are performed on an exercise bike (known in the trade as a cycle ergometer).

On a treadmill, subjects tend to have a slightly higher exercise capacity. Treadmills are bigger and more expensive. Things can get a bit messy if the patient stops suddenly on a moving treadmill, and there tend to be more movement artefacts on the signals recorded.

2.2 Breath-by-breath displays

In the early days of exercise testing, all the air the patient exhaled in a minute was collected in large bag; the gas composition of all the bags was analysed at the end of the test. Faster analysers allow analysis of individual breaths. These breath-by-breath measurements are usually averaged over a few breaths, to smooth the graphs out. In the example shown in Figure 2.1, ventilation increases during exercise; although this is a 'breath-by-breath' plot, there are only about five points per minute because the computer has averaged several breaths to give a smoother plot.

2.3 Incremental or constant workload?

For exploring a particular physiological question in an experiment or assessing the effects of an intervention, a steady state CPEX protocol may be chosen. This means setting a workload and keeping it constant throughout the test—the subject just keeps going for as long as they can. If the workload is too low or the subject is fitter than expected, the test could go on for a long time (unless the subject quits because of boredom, in which case the physiological data is less informative).

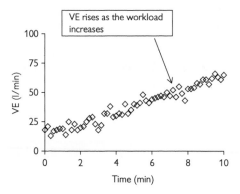

Fig. 2.1 Breath-by-breath plot showing minute ventilation (VE) rising during a CPEX. Each point is the average of several breaths.

It is much more common to gradually increase the workload to the maximum that the subject can perform. The rate at which the ramp increases is chosen so that the test should last about 10 min.

2.4 **End points**

Most of the time, the patient will continue until they are unable to cycle any longer. This is called a symptom-limited maximal exercise test. At the point when they stop, they grade their symptoms using a Borg or visual analogue scale.

> Learning point
>
> *Most CPEX results will be breath-by-breath plots of a symptom-limited maximum test, during which the workload is steadily increased until the subject can no longer keep turning the cycle ergometer.*

2.5 **Measurements**

After ensuring that the equipment is calibrated and working correctly, the bike is adjusted to suit the patient and the procedure is explained to the subject, who is then connected to the monitoring equipment. After a mouthpiece or mask is attached to the subject, measurements can commence.

2.5.1 **Resting baseline**

Just putting a mask over the face can alter the breathing pattern, so a minute or two is allowed for this to stabilize so that there is a stable resting baseline.

2.5.2 **Unloaded cycling**

Once the subject starts to turn the pedals of the ergometer, there will be another change in their breathing pattern as they anticipate having to perform additional muscular work. Again, it takes a minute or two for this to stabilize.

2.5.3 **Increasing the workload**

It is now time to slowly increase the workload. As the resistance gets harder and harder, at some stage the subject will be unable to keep the pedals turning at the required rate, and they will have to stop. It is important to record what forced the subject to stop, how their legs and breathing felt, and whether they had any other symptoms.

2.5.4 **Recovery**

After removing the workload, the subject should continue with a couple of minutes of unloaded cycling as a 'warm down'; this will help prevent any sudden fall in blood pressure. It is worth monitoring the electrocardiogram (ECG) for a few minutes after the test: very occasionally informative changes develop during this recovery period. If after about 10 min or so the subject feels back to their normal self, they can be disconnected from the monitoring and allowed to leave.

2.6 **Graphical displays**

2.6.1 **Phases of the CPEX**

On the graphs displayed during the test and on the reports generated subsequently, there are often vertical lines to delineate the different phases of the test. One of the most popular displays has nine graphs on a page. The graph shown in Figure 2.2 is usually top left in a nine-panel display.

So that the plots don't become too cluttered, the vertical lines will be omitted from subsequent graphs in this book: in all examples the load starts at time zero, with the resting and unloaded phases starting at -4 and -2 min respectively.

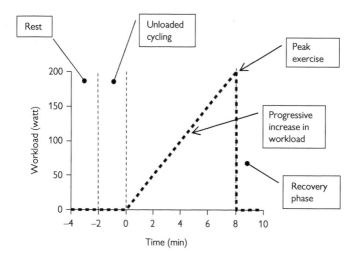

Fig. 2.2 Workload during a CPEX, showing the different phases of the test.

Practical tip

The workload-vs-time plot will help identification of the different phases of CPEX graphs when they are presented in an unfamiliar format.

2.6.2 **Predicted values and ranges**

On CPEX graphs which have a single horizontal line, this is probably the predicted value. Two horizontal lines are sometimes used for the upper and lower limits of normal for a CPEX parameter. With the vertical lines for the phases of the test, the plot starts to look more like a grid for a game of noughts-and-crosses.

The plots in this book have been kept as simple as possible: no vertical lines, generally only one Y-axis, and usually just one horizontal line to show the predicted value (Figure 2.3). The principles learnt can then be applied to a multicoloured nine-panel display. When there are two parameters on the same graph, the axis labels, plot, and horizontal line(s) for predicted values will all be in the same colour.

During a CPEX, the scale of the graphs change several times during the test. Quite a small rise in heart rate (HR), for example, can look like a normal rise on the final printed plots (Figure 2.4); careful examination of the scale shows it only goes up to 100.

Practical tip

Always check the numbers on the Y-axis of a CPEX plot: some computerized systems will 'autoscale' the graph to fill the whole plot.

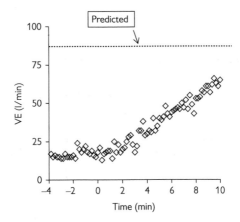

Fig. 2.3 VE rising during a CPEX but falling short of the level predicted for maximum exercise.

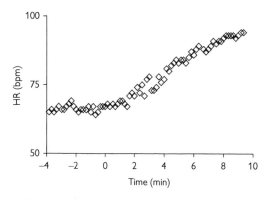

Fig. 2.4 HR during a CPEX, with a small rise exaggerated by the scale on the Y-axis.

Physiology

Workload

'Watts' (W) are sometimes used as the X-axis on CPEX graphs. Basically, this represents the work done against the resistance of the treadmill, which will increase steadily with the load in an incremental test.

A watt is a joule-per-second. Joules, like calories, are units of energy. If the volume of oxygen (O_2) taken in by the subject is known, it is possible to then calculate how efficient the subject is, i.e. how much external work is done for every millilitre of O_2 taken in. In clinical practice, this sort of calculation seldom yields particularly useful information. For simplicity, most of the graphs in this book use 'Time' on the X-axis.

Another unit sometimes used is the 'MET'. This expresses the work done as a multiple of the resting metabolic expenditure, which is assumed to be 3.5 ml O_2 kg/min. The MET is used as a way of giving a rough estimate of VO_2 from the work done on an exercise bike or treadmill in a gym, with no direct respiratory measurements.

2.7 **Supervising a CPEX**

Practical tip

Supervising a CPEX is more informative than simply reviewing the printed results.

Almost all exercise tests continue until the subject decides to stop, but there are a few occasions when you should stop the test early. Absolute indications to stop a test are largely cardiac and won't come as a surprise. (It goes without saying that standard resuscitation equipment should be available during a CPEX).

2.7.1 **Dysrhythmias**

Patients with heart disease may have some ectopics at rest, which will often disappear on exercise. It is more worrying if ventricular ectopics start to occur in pairs or triplets, or if there is a change in their morphology. It will usually be prudent to stop at this stage. Once short runs of ventricular tachycardia develop, the test should definitely be terminated. If atrial fibrillation develops during the test, then this is a good explanation for the patient's symptoms; and there is little point in continuing with the test.

Ventricular ectopics which are present on the resting ECG often disappear on exercise. If they start to occur in runs, stop the CPEX.

2.7.2 **ST segment changes**

If clear ST segment depression of 2 mm or more develops during the test, myocardial ischaemia is present, and there is little point in pushing the patient any further. To some extent, this will depend on the circumstances of the patient and the reason for the test. If a patient with undiagnosed breathlessness develops ST segment depression, then a diagnosis of myocardial ischaemia can be made and the test stopped. However, continuing the test a little longer could be acceptable and informative in a patient who is borderline for potentially curative cancer surgery and is known to have angina.

Myocardial ischaemia is quite a common diagnosis for the sorts of people who attend for a CPEX, as they will have reported breathlessness but will have reasonable lung function and X-rays (or are being worked up for surgery). The O_2 pulse can be used as a proxy of cardiac output, which may fall towards the end of exercise if the myocardium becomes ischaemic. This will be discussed in more detail later.

2.7.3 **Oxygen desaturation**

Desaturation during a CPEX is uncommon, except when exercising patients with known lung disease (for example, prior to an intervention). There are no absolute thresholds, but for a diagnostic CPEX, if the SpO_2 was normal at rest, then the test should be stopped if it starts to fall below 90%. (It usually goes a bit lower before starting to rise again).

Falling SpO_2 during exercise suggests significant pathology. However, saturations detected by finger probe can fall if the subject grips the handlebars tightly. When desaturation occurs during exercise, the patient should be asked to relax their grip on the bars. (An earlobe sensor is obviously not liable to this problem). If the SpO_2 jumps up quickly, then the desaturation was an artefact: real falls in SpO_2 recover slowly when the subject stops exercising.

2.7.4 **Blood pressure**

Systolic blood pressure should rise progressively during exercise. If it starts to fall, it probably means that the subject is developing significant myocardial ischaemia.

2.7.5 **Airflow limitation**

CPEX equipment that displays flow-volume plots can be used to detect expiratory airflow limitation. It should be looked for at intervals during the test, being indicated by a concave 'scalloping' of the expiratory loop. This will be considered in more detail in Chapter 6.

Exercise-induced asthma

Most CPEX protocols also require that the patient's forced expiratory volume in 1 s (FEV$_1$) is recorded at two or three time points after stopping exercise. This is intended to detect a fall in FEV$_1$ related to exercise-induced asthma. The pick-up rate is low because exercise-related bronchospasm is largely caused by airway dehydration and cooling rather than circulating mediators released by exercise itself.

A fall in FEV$_1$ of 20% or more during the 10 min or so after a CPEX is a strong pointer to the diagnosis of exercise-induced asthma, but this diagnosis is not excluded if the FEV$_1$ doesn't fall.

Further reading

Balady GJ, Arena R, Sietsema K, Myers J, Coke L, Fletcher GF, et al. Clinician's guide to cardiopulmonary exercise testing in adults: a scientific statement from the American Heart Association. Circulation. 2010 Jul 13;122(2):191–225. PubMed PMID: 20585013.

Hansen JE, Sue DY, Wasserman K. Predicted values for clinical exercise testing. Am Rev Respir Dis. 1984 Feb;129(2 Pt 2):S49–55. PubMed PMID: 6421218.

Neder JA, Nery LE, Peres C, Whipp BJ. Reference values for dynamic responses to incremental cycle ergometry in males and females aged 20 to 80. Am J Respir Crit Care Med. 2001 Oct 15;164(8 Pt 1):1481–6. PubMed PMID: 11704600.

Part 2

Key cardiopulmonary exercise test parameters

Chapter 3

Oxygen uptake

> **Key points**
> - Maximum oxygen uptake (VO_2max) is the single most important cardiopulmonary exercise test (CPEX) parameter.
> - A VO_2max less than 80% of predicted is abnormal.
> - The lower the VO_2max, the worse the outcome.

3.1 What is oxygen uptake?

Oxygen (O_2) uptake is the volume of oxygen (VO_2) utilized in metabolism by the body, primarily in mitochondria. It is the difference between inhaled and exhaled O_2 fractions and is expressed as ml/min or standardized for weight as ml kg/min.

3.2 How is it measured?

A mouthpiece or mask is attached to the subject, in order to see the volume of air they breathe in and out. The percentage of O_2 in the inspired air is 21%. The amount of O_2 remaining in the exhaled air can be measured by passing it through an O_2 analyser. It is then easy to calculate the volume of O_2 that has been used by the body.

> **Physiology**
>
> Cellular respiration
>
> *Just a quick reminder of what respiration is all about. For muscles to contract they need energy, which they get by burning fuel. Carbohydrate is the fuel, which is 'burnt' using O_2. Carbon dioxide (CO_2) and water (H_2O) are produced as waste products.*
>
> $$Fuel + O_2 \rightarrow CO_2 + H_2O + ENERGY$$
>
> *When glucose is the substrate, the chemical equation is:*
>
> $$C_6H_{12}O_6 + 6\,O_2 \rightarrow 6\,CO_2 + 6\,H_2O + ENERGY$$
>
> *Notice that, for this substrate, the amount of O_2 used and CO_2 are the same:*
>
> $$6\,O_2 \rightarrow 6\,CO_2$$
>
> *This is a respiratory quotient of 1. If fat is the substrate, the ratio is less than 1.0, with less CO_2 produced than O_2 used up.*

3.3 **VO$_2$max**

The highest value that the VO$_2$ reaches during an exercise test is termed the VO$_2$max. This may also be referred to as the *peak* VO$_2$ or aerobic capacity. It isn't quite the same as the *maximal* VO$_2$, which is the highest value that could be attained by the individual rather than that actually measured. On a nine-panel display, VO$_2$ vs time (or load) is usually top right (Figure 3.1).

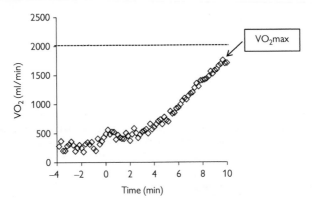

Fig. 3.1. VO$_2$ rising during a symptom-limited CPEX. VO$_2$max is the highest value reached.

3.4 **What determines VO$_2$max?**

VO$_2$max is influenced by age and gender, and to a lesser extent, height. To work out what a subject should have achieved in terms of a VO$_2$max, data from several studies can be combined in a regression analysis to create an equation for a predicted value (see Figure 3.2). An example derived from five studies (see Cooper and Storer, in the Bibliography) for a male would be:

$$VO_2 \ max(ml \ kg/min) = 50 - (0.4 \times age \ in \ years).$$

To get to ml/min, multiply by ideal body weight (which is 71.6 × height in metres − 51.8). This will be done automatically by the CPEX computer.

3.5 **Tables**

Although graphs give some idea of how close a subject got to the predicted, the results really need to be tabulated (Table 3.1).

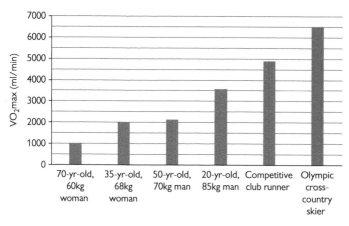

Fig. 3.2 Examples of VO$_2$max seen with different subjects on a cycle ergometer.

Table 3.1 Measured and predicted values for oxygen uptake at peak exercise (VO$_2$max) in an individual undergoing a cardiopulmonary exercise test. VO$_2$max is greater than 80% of predicted, so is within the normal range for this individual.

	Measured (ml/min)	% predicted
VO$_2$max	2006	92

A cut-off of 80% predicted is widely used to define normality in a CPEX. The problem with this approach is that it implies that the larger the value that is predicted, the more variable normal results are likely to be. Using per cent predicted also does not take into consideration that the amount of variation in normal individuals is influenced significantly by sex, age, and height; that is to say, a group of young but small men may have the same predicted VO$_2$max as older, taller men (or taller women of the same age), but the variation in VO$_2$max in each group may be quite different.

An alternative is to use centile tables, such as those of the American College of Sports Medicine (ACSM; see Further reading). These are split by sex and height into five-year age bands, from 20 to 79 years. Being in the bottom 20% is usually referred to as 'poor performance', whereas being in the bottom 5% (below the 5th centile, if you prefer) is classified as 'abnormal'. For the moment, the 80% rule will suffice, despite its shortcomings.

Learning point

A VO$_2$max greater than 80% predicted means that it is very unlikely that the subject has clinically significant pathology affecting their heart or lungs.

Clinical scenario

Normal VO$_2$max

What happens when a patient with shortness of breath on exercise has a normal VO$_2$max? Most of the time, they find it reassuring that there is nothing seriously wrong. There may be a slight worry that their VO$_2$max has fallen from a higher value, even although it is still within the normal range at this point. Even if there is something going on, it is at a fairly early stage, and delaying treatment for a while is unlikely to be detrimental. Probably the best thing to do is wait and see: to review the patient in a few months and consider repeating the CPEX. An exercise programme during the intervening period would be a good idea.

3.6 **What causes a low VO$_2$max?**

A low VO$_2$max (Figure 3.3) requires explanation, and much of the rest of this book will be spent looking at ways of working this out (Box 3.1).

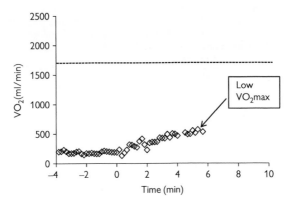

Fig. 3.3 VO$_2$ during a CPEX, with VO$_2$max falling well short of the predicted value.

Box 3.1 A few reasons for a low VO$_2$max

- The subject stopped before they were at their physiological maximum exercise capacity, perhaps because they didn't try hard enough or because of something like pain from arthritic joints.
- The subject is unfit, and their maximum exercise capacity is less than it should be.
- The subject has heart disease, so the circulation couldn't get enough O$_2$ to the muscles.
- The subject has lung disease, with insufficient capacity to get O$_2$ into the lungs, or from the lungs into the blood.

3.7 How to express VO₂max: ml/min or ml kg/min?

The best way to express VO_2max is in ml/min. Unfortunately, much of the data on VO_2max as a predictive tool uses ml kg/min. In patients with a lot of peripheral oedema, their 'dry' weight should be estimated; otherwise, VO_2max in ml kg/min will be falsely low. (In other words, the VO_2 value in ml/min is divided by too many kilograms, giving a falsely low result). Similarly, in a very obese subject, lean body mass should be estimated, using skin calipers, etc. In practice, the value is often just left as ml kg/min. For example, Table 3.2 is an extract from the ACSM table, giving the expected values for VO_2max in a 50–59-year-old sedentary physician. Only one per cent of the population in this age group would be expected to have a VO_2max less than 21 ml kg/min, so a value of 20 ml kg/min would clearly be abnormal.

Table 3.2 Distribution of maximum oxygen intake (VO_2max) in a normal population of 50–59-year-old males.

VO₂max (ml kg/min)	54	47	43	41	38	37	35	33	31	28	26	21
% of normal population below this VO₂max	99	90	80	70	60	50	40	30	20	10	5	1

Learning point

A VO_2max of less than 20 ml kg/min is low; less than 15 ml kg/min is moderate impairment of cardiorespiratory function; less than 10 ml kg/min is severe impairment.

3.8 VO₂max, gender, and age

Returning to the ACSM tables, Table 3.3 shows the 5% cut-off values for different ages in males and females. In other words, only 5% of the normal population would be expected to have a VO_2max below this value: a result such as this would classify the subject as 'abnormal'. A VO_2max of 20 ml kg/min is clearly abnormal for a 20-year-old man, but is pretty normal for a 70-year-old man or 60-year-old woman.

Table 3.3 Lower limit of normal for maximum oxygen uptake (VO_2max) in different age groups.

Age (years)	VO₂max (ml kg/min) Males	Females
20–29	32.3	26.4
30–39	31.1	25.5
40–49	29.4	24.1
50–59	25.8	21.9
60–69	22.1	20.1
70–79	19.3	17.9

The expected normal value for VO$_2$max is less in females than males and declines with age.

3.9 **VO$_2$max and mortality**

Many studies have investigated the ability of VO$_2$max to predict adverse outcomes, especially in patients at high risk of complications or death. Three main findings from these studies are apparent:

1. Lower VO$_2$max is associated with earlier death in the general population without diagnosed major illness.

2. VO$_2$max is closely related to risk of death or major complication in cardiac and lung surgery and is associated to varying degrees with poor outcomes in other major surgeries.

3. Lower VO$_2$max is associated with a poorer outcome in chronic cardiopulmonary diseases.

Further reading

Bassett DR, Jr., Howley ET. Limiting factors for maximum oxygen uptake and determinants of endurance performance. Med Sci Sports Exerc. 2000 Jan;32(1):70–84. PubMed PMID: 10647532.

Hill AV, Lupton H. Muscular exercise, lactic acid, and utilization of oxygen. Q.J.Med 1923 16:135–71.

Mora S, Redberg RF, Cui Y, Whiteman MK, Flaws JA, Sharrett AR, et al. Ability of exercise testing to predict cardiovascular and all-cause death in asymptomatic women: a 20-year follow-up of the lipid research clinics prevalence study. JAMA. 2003 Sep 24;290(12):1600–7. PubMed PMID: 14506119.

Neder JA, Dal Corso S, Malaguti C, Reis S, De Fuccio MB, Schmidt H, et al. The pattern and timing of breathing during incremental exercise: a normative study. Eur Respir J. 2003 Mar;21(3):530–8. PubMed PMID: 12662013.

Whipp BJ. Dynamics of pulmonary gas exchange. Circulation. 1987 Dec;76(6 Pt 2):VI18–28. PubMed PMID: 3119250.

Chapter 4

Heart rate

> **Key points**
> - Normal subjects will reach 80% or more of their predicted maximum heart rate (HR): cardiac output is what determines their exercise capacity.
> - Unfit subjects and patients with heart disease will also reach 80% of predicted maximum HR, but their maximum oxygen uptake (VO_2max) will be low.
> - If the maximum HR is low, either the subject didn't try very hard or something other than the heart is limiting exercise capacity.

4.1 **Normal HR response**

During a cardiopulmonary exercise test (CPEX), HR usually increases steadily during the test, and is highest at the point where the subject stops the test (Figure 4.1). This graph is in the middle of the top row on a nine-panel display.

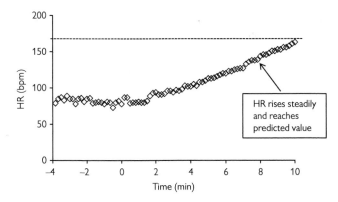

Fig. **4.1** HR rising steadily during a CPEX; bpm, beats per minute.

On a CPEX summary report, the subject's maximum HR can be compared with the predicted value (Table 4.1). The maximum HR can be predicted fairly reliably using the equation:

$$\text{Maximum HR bpm} = 220 - \text{age (in years)}.$$

Table 4.1 Measured and predicted values for maximum oxygen uptake (VO_2) and heart rate (HR) in an individual undergoing a cardiopulmonary exercise test.

Peak exercise:		
	Measured	% predicted
VO_2 (ml/min)	2006	92
HR (bpm)	178	90

HR is the factor which limits exercise capacity in normal subjects (and those with heart disease), i.e. the subject will attain their predicted HR at maximal exercise. Reaching 80% of the predicted rate is usually considered normal.

> **Learning point**
>
> At peak exercise, a normal subject **should** reach 80% or more of their predicted maximum HR.

4.2 **Low HR reserve**

An HR >80% predicted at peak exercise is often referred to as a low HR reserve, i.e. the possibility of increasing HR any further is pretty limited. A normal subject will attain at least 80% of their predicted HR at peak exercise, and, of course, their VO_2max will be normal. Unfit subjects will push up their HR pretty quickly, as will those with impaired left ventricular function in whom the only way to get more cardiac output is by increasing their HR (Figure 4.2). This is also seen in those with pulmonary vascular disease in whom right ventricular output is impaired. (All these subjects will have a low VO_2max.)

> **Practical tip**
>
> Don't stop a CPEX just because the subject has reached their predicted HR: keep going until they have to stop because of symptoms (unless, of course, they develop dysrhythmias, etc).

4.3 **High HR reserve**

The HR will not reach 80% predicted (i.e. there will be a high HR reserve) if the subject stops early, as would be the case if they stopped after 7 min in the first example in this chapter (Figure 4.3).

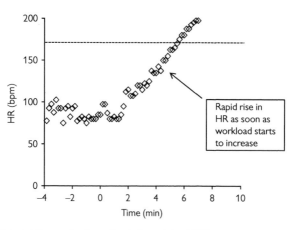

Fig. 4.2 Rapid rise in HR exceeding the predicted value early in a CPEX.

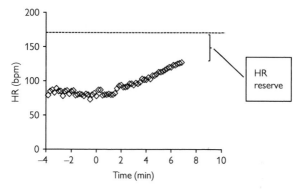

Fig. 4.3 HR during a sub-maximal CPEX, showing the presence of a significant HR reserve at the point the subject stopped.

In tabular form, these results would look like Table 4.2.

A high HR reserve (i.e. HR not reaching 80% of predicted) occurs when, from the heart's point of view, the test was stopped too early. In addition to sub-maximal effort, a high HR reserve is seen when exercise is limited by something other than cardiac function. Examples of this would be lung disease or peripheral vascular disease.

Practical tip
'Did the subject fail to reach 80% or more of their predicted HR?' and 'Was there an abnormally high HR reserve?' are the same question.

Table 4.2 Results from a cardiopulmonary exercise test in an individual who made a sub-maximal effort. Neither value reaches 80% of predicted.

Peak exercise:		
	Measured	% predicted
VO_2 (ml/min)	1258	64
HR (bpm)	111	58

Clinical scenario

Chronotropic insufficiency

Chronotropic insufficiency is a fancy way of saying that the HR doesn't rise normally (Figure 4.4). Since cardiac output is stroke volume × HR, the ability of the heart to increase its output (and hence the volume of oxygen (O_2) it transports from the lungs) will be compromised. Drugs such as beta-blockers may be the culprit or sinoatrial node dysfunction. This pattern is not particularly common, but worth looking out for.

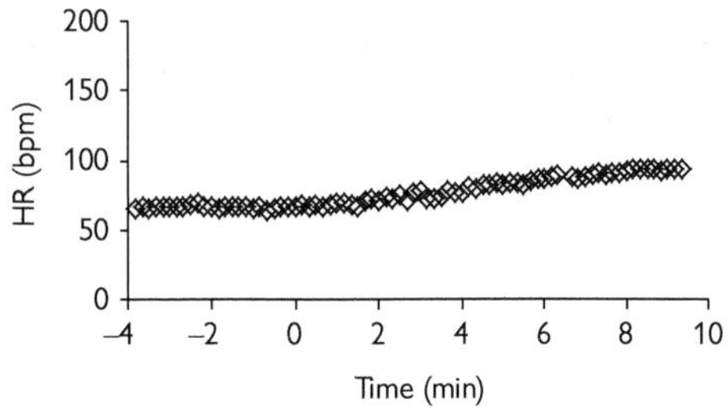

Fig. 4.4 Low rise in HR during a CPEX. This is sometimes called 'chronotropic insufficiency'.

4.4 High HR

It is not uncommon to see a high HR in an anxious patient, although this will often settle at the beginning of exercise and then rise in a normal pattern subsequently (Figure 4.5). A persistent tachycardia may indicate poor ventricular function: since stroke volume cannot increase, the only way of pushing up cardiac output is by a faster HR.

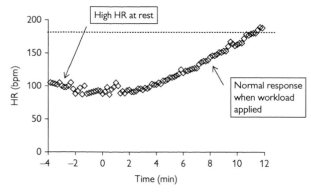

Fig. 4.5 Slightly high resting HR, but normal rise during loaded cycling.

Further reading

Ellestad MH, Wan MK. Predictive implications of stress testing. Follow-up of 2700 subjects after maximum treadmill stress testing. Circulation. 1975 Feb;51(2):363–9. PubMed PMID: 1112017.

Jouven X, Empana JP, Schwartz PJ, Desnos M, Courbon D, Ducimetiere P. Heart-rate profile during exercise as a predictor of sudden death. N Engl J Med. 2005 May 12;352(19):1951–8. PubMed PMID: 15888695.

Chapter 5

Oxygen pulse

> ## Key points
> - Oxygen (O_2) pulse can be used as an indirect indicator of cardiac stroke volume.
> - A normal subject should achieve an O_2 pulse of more than 10 ml/beat at peak exercise.
> - A plateau in the O_2 pulse at a low value implies limited cardiac output, because of either heart disease or disorders of the pulmonary circulation.
> - Don't over-interpret a low O_2 pulse, particularly if the maximum oxygen uptake (VO_2max) is normal.

5.1 What is the O_2 pulse?

The O_2 pulse is simply oxygen uptake (VO_2) divided by heart rate (HR):

$$O_2 \text{ pulse (ml/beat)} = VO_2 \text{ (ml/min) / HR (beats per minute (bpm))}.$$

5.2 What does the O_2 pulse measure?

The O_2 pulse is the amount of O_2 taken up by the lungs into the blood with each heartbeat. If there is more blood flowing through the lungs, then more O_2 will be taken up. Cardiac output is the product of HR and stroke volume, so VO_2 is related to cardiac output by the equation:

$$\text{cardiac output} = \text{stroke volume} \times \text{HR} \approx VO_2$$

By rearranging these terms, the O_2 pulse becomes:

$$O_2 \text{ pulse} = VO_2 \text{ / HR} \approx \text{stroke volume}.$$

> ### Learning point
> *The O_2 pulse can be used as an indirect indicator of cardiac stroke volume.*

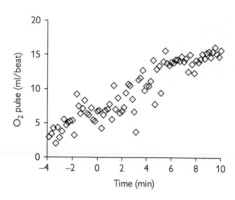

Fig. 5.1 The O$_2$ pulse rising during the early part of a cardiopulmonary exercise test.

The O$_2$ pulse is usually plotted on the same graph as the HR. In a normal subject, the O$_2$ pulse increases during the early part of the test, as stroke volume increases, then tends to tail off—any further increase in cardiac output (and hence VO$_2$) is related to increasing HR (Figure 5.1).

5.3 **Normal values**

Predicted values for the O$_2$ pulse at peak exercise can be derived by dividing the predicted VO$_2$max by the predicted maximum HR. For example, if VO$_2$max is predicted to be 3600 ml/min and maximum HR 180 bpm, then the O$_2$ pulse should be 20 ml/ beat. As with many other cardiopulmonary exercise test (CPEX) parameters, 80% is used as the cut-off for abnormally low values (16 ml/beat in this example). As a rule of thumb, the O$_2$ pulse will generally reach at least 10 ml/beat in a normal subject, and often 15 ml/beat or more.

> **Learning point**
>
> *A normal subject should achieve an O$_2$ pulse of at least 10 ml/beat during a CPEX.*

5.4 **Low O$_2$ pulse**

In heart disease, stroke volume may not increase at all. The only way to increase cardiac output is by speeding the heart up. In this case, the O$_2$ pulse (i.e. stroke volume) will remain much the same throughout the test (Figure 5.2).

If the subject develops cardiac ischaemia, stroke volume will be suddenly impaired (Figure 5.3). Sometimes you will see this before any electrocardiogram (ECG) changes.

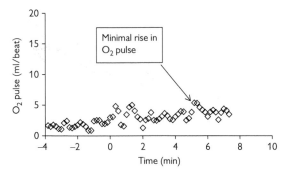

Fig. 5.2 Failure of O_2 pulse to rise during a CPEX in a subject with poor left ventricular function.

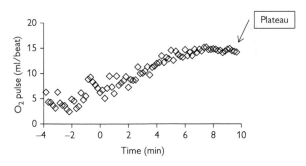

Fig. 5.3 Plateau in the O_2 pulse with the development of myocardial ischaemia and left ventricular dysfunction.

Learning point

If the O_2 pulse reaches a plateau, suspect impairment of cardiac output (due to heart disease or pulmonary vascular disease), particularly if the peak value is less than 10 ml/beat.

Clinical scenario

The O_2 pulse in athletes
One of the distinguishing features of a fit individual is their ability to achieve a very high O_2 pulse. They do this mainly by increasing cardiac stroke volume, but they also increase the size of the capillaries in their peripheral muscles. This latter process allows them to extract more O_2 from the blood, which leaves more room for O_2 to be taken up in the lungs. (In other words, there is a larger difference in O_2 content between mixed-venous blood entering the lungs and arterial blood leaving them). More VO_2 for the same pulse rate leads to a larger O_2 pulse. Elite athletes can achieve 40 ml/beat or more.

Physiology

The Fick equation

*The Fick equation states that VO_2 is the product of cardiac output multiplied by the difference between the O_2 **content** of the arterial blood (CaO_2) and that of the mixed venous blood (CvO_2):*

$$VO_2 = Cardiac\ output \times (CaO_2 - CvO_2).$$

The O_2 content depends on the haemoglobin (Hb) concentration and the peripheral oxygen saturation (SpO_2): when fully saturated, one gram of Hb can carry about 1.34 ml of O_2.

If there is arterial O_2 desaturation during a CPEX, as may happen in lung disease or if a foramen ovale opens up, the amount of O_2 taken up by blood in the lungs will be lower. (In other words, there is a smaller difference between the O_2 content of mixed venous blood entering the lungs and that of the poorly-saturated arterial blood leaving the lungs). The O_2 pulse will therefore be low, but not because of a low stroke volume.

Part of the reason that athletes have such a high O_2 pulse is that they are very efficient at extracting O_2 in their muscles, so they achieve a low CvO_2.

Practical tip

There are quite a few things that influence O_2 pulse. Beware of over-interpreting a low peak O_2 pulse (or a plateau), particularly if the VO_2max is normal.

Further reading

Oliveira RB, Myers J, Araujo CG, Arena R, Mandic S, Bensimhon D, et al. Does peak oxygen pulse complement peak oxygen uptake in risk stratifying patients with heart failure? Am J Cardiol. 2009 Aug 15;104(4):554–8. PubMed PMID: 19660611.

Edvardsen E, Hansen BH, Holme IM, Dyrstad SM, Anderssen SA. Reference values for cardiorespiratory response and fitness on the treadmill in a 20–85-year-old population. Chest. 2013 Jan 3. doi: 10.1378/chest.12–1458. [Epub ahead of print]. PubMed PMID: 23287878.

Stringer WW, Hansen JE, Wasserman K. Cardiac output estimated non-invasively from oxygen uptake during exercise. J. Appl. Physiol. 1997. Mar;82(3):908–12. PMID: 9074981

Sun XG, Hansen JE, Oudiz RJ, Wasserman K. Exercise pathophysiology in patients with primary pulmonary hypertension. Circulation. 2001 Jul 24;104(4):429–35. PubMed PMID: 11468205.

Chapter 6

Ventilation

> **Key points**
> - Minute ventilation (VE) increases during a cardiopulmonary test (CPEX).
> - VE does not normally limit exercise.
> - If VE reaches 80% of predicted, this implies there is something wrong with the lungs.
> - Tidal volume (Vt) should increase in the early part of a CPEX.

6.1 **VE**

The measure of ventilation used in an exercise test is *VE*, which is the sum of the volume of all the breaths in one minute. It is the product of the frequency and depth of breathing. In younger subjects, the size of each breath (Vt) will increase three- to fivefold, to about 60% of vital capacity, though this is usually less in older subjects. Frequency of respiration will usually double, though younger and fitter subjects will increase their respiratory rate considerably more.

A normal subject, resting on a cycle ergometer waiting to start a CPEX, might have a respiratory rate of about 12 breaths per minute. With a Vt of, say, 800 ml this would give a VE of just under 10 l/min ($12 \times 0.8 = 9.6$). If the subject is anxious, they may hyperventilate a little in the early phase of a CPEX, but then settle down as the load starts to kick in. This is not unusual, and doesn't imply that their symptoms are due to hyperventilation, particularly if the ventilation rises steadily once they have settled down (Figure 6.1).

6.2 **Predicted values**

Theoretical maximum minute ventilation (VEmax) is usually estimated from a subject's forced expired volume in 1 s (FEV1). The most accurate simple formula seems to be:

$$VEmax = (FEV1 \times 20) + 20$$

with FEV1 in litres and VEmax in litres per minute.

The VEmax a subject is capable of can be assessed by asking them to breathe as deeply and quickly as possible for 15 s and then measuring the amount of gas expired (and quadrupling this value). This is called the maximum voluntary ventilation. However, such manoeuvres are dependent on the motivation of the subject, will lead to hypocapnia, and can provoke bronchoconstriction.

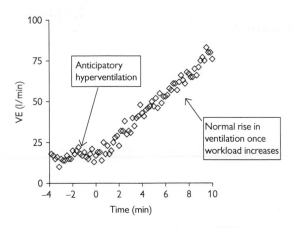

Fig. 6.1 Initial hyperventilation, followed by a normal rise in VE, during a CPEX.

6.3 **Ventilatory reserve**

Ventilatory reserve is the same concept as HR reserve: if VEmax is >80% of the predicted value, then this is called a low ventilatory reserve (i.e. there is little possibility of increasing ventilation any further).

In normal subjects, as well as those with heart disease, cardiac output limits exercise. There is usually sufficient reserve in ventilation that it does not reach 80% of the predicted value (as illustrated by Figure 6.2, Table 6.1).

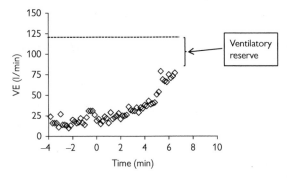

Fig. 6.2 VE rising during a CPEX, but failing to reach the predicted value. The difference between observed and predicted maximum VE is ventilatory reserve.

Table 6.1 Oxygen uptake (VO_2), heart rate (HR) and minute ventilation (VE) at peak exercise in a normal subject undergoing a cardiopulmonary exercise test.

Peak exercise:

	Measured	% predicted
VO_2 (ml/min)	2006	92
HR (bpm)	178	90
VE (l/min)	59	63

Learning point

*Ventilation should **not** reach 80% of predicted during a CPEX in a normal subject.*

6.4 **Ventilatory limitation**

In lung disease, the subject will stop because of ventilatory limitation. From the cardiac point of view, it is as if the patient stopped before maximum capacity was reached, so the HR will be <80% predicted. (Table 6.2)

Table 6.2 Oxygen uptake (VO_2), heart rate (HR), and minute ventilation (VE) at peak exercise in a subject with lung disease undergoing a cardiopulmonary exercise test.

Peak exercise:

	Measured	% predicted
VO_2 (ml/min)	1280	65
HR (bpm)	116	72
VE (l/min)	38	90

Learning point

If VO_2max is low and ventilation exceeds 80% of predicted (i.e. there is a low ventilatory reserve), then there is probably something wrong with the lungs.

In clinical practice, a CPEX doesn't often reveal significant lung disease which could not have been anticipated from the tests you would normally do before resorting to a diagnostic CPEX. Nevertheless, it is important to be able to recognize the sorts of abnormalities seen when the lungs are the factor limiting exercise, particularly when looking at lots of tests prior to thoracic surgery or pulmonary rehabilitation programmes.

Practical tip

Trained athletes can push themselves well beyond the predicted VO₂max. Their stroke volume is such that they can increase their cardiac output considerably, so they continue to exercise for longer and stray into the region where they reach predicted ventilation. This does not imply that there is anything wrong with their lungs.

6.5 **Vt**

In a normal subject, Vt increases during low-intensity exercise. As the load gets more severe, further increases in ventilation are achieved by increasing the rate (Figure 6.3).

Looking at the Vt/VE plot, if ventilation increases without much rise in Vt, then this must be because the frequency of breathing increases. Patients with lung disease tend to have a flatter Vt/VE plot, i.e. they reach this plateau much earlier. They rely on increasing rate more than Vt (Figure 6.4).

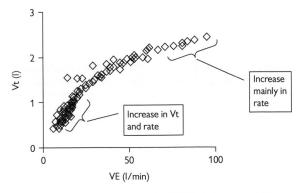

Fig. 6.3 Increase in Vt and VE during the early phase of a CPEX. In the later stages, VE increases with little change in Vt (i.e. the increase is mainly due to rising respiratory rate).

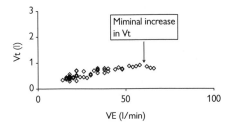

Fig. 6.4 Failure of Vt to increase during a CPEX, implying the presence of lung disease.

Clinical scenario

Dysfunctional breathing

Looking at the VE/time (Figure 6.5) and Vt/VE (Figure 6.6) plots can give some clues that a subject's breathlessness is a problem of perception, rather than indicating a physiological problem with the heart or lungs. Rather erratic ventilation implies 'dysfunctional breathing', which is probably a better term than 'hyperventilation syndrome'. This will be discussed in more detail when looking at the relationship between ventilation and carbon dioxide (CO_2) output in later chapters.

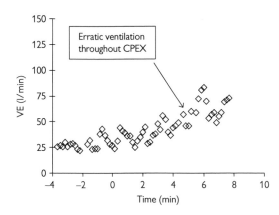

Fig. 6.5 Irregular increase in VE during a CPEX, implying dysfunctional breathing with psychological rather than physiological factors influencing ventilation.

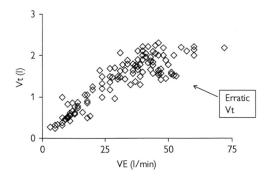

Fig. 6.6 Wide scatter of Vt implying dysfunctional breathing.

Physiology

Airflow limitation

Many CPEX systems can plot flow-volume loops for each breath during the test. At low levels of exercise, this loop will look smooth and convex. As exercise progresses, the expiratory limb starts to become concave. If the maximum flow-volume loop (recorded before the start of the CPEX test) is superimposed, then it can be seen that the only way to increase flow is to move left along the volume axis. Someone with severe airflow obstruction who is already hyperinflated will have nowhere to go (in terms of increasing their lung volume, that is): they cannot increase flow to exhale a larger Vt, and they cannot afford to shorten expiration in order to increase respiratory rate. Their ventilation is limited, and they will be forced to stop the test because of breathlessness (Figure 6.7).

With age, loss of elasticity in the lungs means that the airways are more prone to collapse during expiration. This probably explains why older subjects don't push their Vt quite as high as younger subjects: they can't get as much air out before it's time for the next breath.

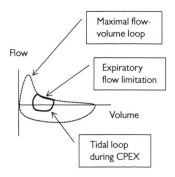

Fig. 6.7 Expiratory limitation of flow during a CPEX.

Further reading

Loveridge B, West P, Kryger MH, Anthonisen NR. Alteration in breathing pattern with progression of chronic obstructive pulmonary disease. Am Rev Respir Dis. 1986 Nov;134(5):930–4. PubMed PMID: 3777689.

Neder JA, Dal Corso S, Malaguti C, Reis S, De Fuccio MB, Schmidt H, et al. The pattern and timing of breathing during incremental exercise: a normative study. Eur Respir J. 2003 Mar;21(3):530–8. PubMed PMID: 12662013.

Carbon dioxide output

- Carbon dioxide (CO_2) output increases during exercise.
- CO_2 is produced by burning fuel.
- CO_2 is also a by-product of buffering lactic acid.
- Exhaled CO_2 comes from alveolar ventilation.

7.1 What is CO_2 output?

Carbon dioxide output (VCO_2) is the volume of carbon dioxide exhaled, expressed in ml/min.

7.2 How is VCO_2 measured?

The amount of oxygen taken in by the body (VO_2) is calculated by looking at how much oxygen (O_2) is left in the expired air. Working out VCO_2 is just as simple: there is no CO_2 in the inspired air, so looking at the concentration in expired air and multiplying it by the minute ventilation (VE) yields VCO_2 in ml/min. This is an additional plot on the graph, usually placed in the top right-hand corner of the nine-panel display, alongside VO_2 (Figure 7.1).

Physiology

Where does the CO_2 come from?
For the purposes of interpreting a CPEX, there are two important sources of CO_2. Firstly, from metabolism of fuel to produce energy:

$$C_6H_{12}O_6 + 6\,O_2 \rightarrow 6\,CO_2 + 6\,H_2O + ENERGY$$

Secondly, when the hydrogen ions (H^+) from lactic acid are buffered by bicarbonate (HCO_3), the result is water (H_2O) and CO_2. Anaerobic metabolism will be discussed in more detail in due course, but for the moment just note that CO_2 pops up in the right hand side of this equation:

$$H^+ + HCO_3^- \rightarrow H_2O + CO_2$$

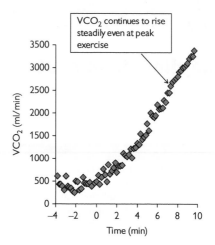

Fig. 7.1 VCO_2 increasing during a cardiopulmonary exercise test (CPEX).

> **Learning point**
>
> *During a CPEX, CO_2 comes from burning fuel in O_2 (aerobic metabolism) and from buffering the H^+ from lactic acid (generated by anaerobic metabolism).*

7.3 **Ventilation and VCO_2**

The link between alveolar ventilation and VCO_2 is pretty tight: more alveolar ventilation means more VCO_2 (Figure 7.2). Lots of ventilation without much VCO_2 implies that the lungs aren't working. One way of looking at this is to plot VE against VCO_2, but it's probably easier to assess the efficiency of ventilation by looking at ventilatory equivalents (VEq; see Chapter 10) (Figure 7.1).

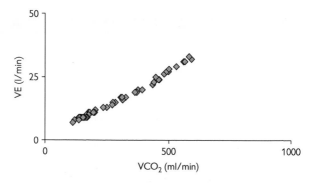

Fig. 7.2 VE is closely linked to VCO_2 during a CPEX.

Physiology

Alveolar ventilation

There are two types of dead space (Vd). Anatomical dead space volume just means the volume of the conducting airways, which **can't** participate in gas exchange because they aren't alveoli.

Physiological Vd is the volume of the lung which **doesn't** participate in gas exchange, either because it is anatomical Vd or because the alveoli aren't perfused (Figure 7.3).

During exercise, Vd declines a bit as more lung units are recruited. Vt increases, as we've seen, so Vd/Vt falls. Some CPEX reports will give you numerical values for this index. It is usually about 0.4, but decreases to 0.2 during exercise.

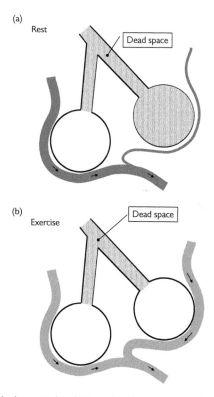

(a) Rest

Dead space

(b) Exercise

Dead space

Fig. 7.3 'Physiological' dead space, i.e. lung that is ventilated but does not participate in gas exchange, decreases on exercise. As cardiac output rises, blood flow through under-perfused lung units (on the right in this figure) increases, and ventilation-perfusion matching becomes more even.

7.4 **Acidaemia and ventilation**

Extreme exercise will result in anaerobic metabolism, and the production of lactic acid will eventually swamp the buffering mechanisms. When this happens, more acid appears in the blood: this is called acidaemia.

Acidaemia stimulates ventilation, as for example in patients with diabetic ketoacidosis or renal failure. This hyperventilation in response to acidosis can often be seen on the VE/VCO_2 plot (Figure 7.4), and the point at which it starts is called the respiratory compensation point (RCP; beyond which there is respiratory compensation for acidaemia).

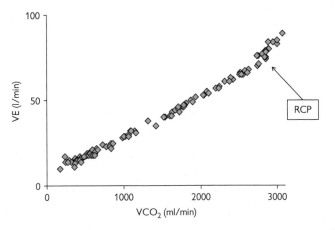

Fig. **7.4** Increase in VE out of proportion to change in VCO_2 beyond the RCP, when acidaemia starts to stimulate ventilation.

7.5 **Hypercapnia and hypocapnia**

Carbon dioxide diffuses pretty quickly out of the blood into the alveolar gas. Unlike O_2, which is much less soluble, it is not particularly affected by processes such as fibrosis, which thicken the alveolar wall.

The arterial CO_2 level ($PaCO_2$) is the driving pressure, which determines how fast CO_2 flows out into the alveolar gas—if a subject hyperventilates and lowers their $PaCO_2$, then the driving pressure is lower and less CO_2 will be exhaled. This explains the change in slope beyond the RCP.

If the $PaCO_2$ is high, then the driving pressure is high, and more CO_2 will be exhaled for a given level of ventilation. In practice, the possibility of hypercapnic respiratory failure is likely to have been picked up earlier on in the diagnostic process, prior to a CPEX.

7.6 **VE/VCO$_2$ and mortality**

Curiously, several studies have shown that VE/VCO_2 is a surprisingly good predictor of subsequent morbidity and mortality, especially in patients with heart failure. A high VE/

VCO_2 implies that there is a lot of ventilation wasted on dead space, possibly because of poor perfusion of some areas in the lungs, which are unable therefore to participate in gas exchange.

Another explanation for a high VE/VCO_2 might be a low $PaCO_2$, hence reducing the driving pressure to get CO_2 from the blood out into the alveolar gas. Patients with severe heart failure sometimes have a low $PaCO_2$, probably because they hyperventilate in order to try and keep their arterial O_2 level (PaO_2) up. A low $PaCO_2$ is associated with the development of Cheyne-Stokes respiration, which is a very poor prognostic sign in heart failure, particularly if seen during wakefulness.

Physiology

Control of breathing

Breathing is pretty unusual in that it has voluntary and involuntary control. A degree of hyperventilation is not unusual in the early phases of a CPEX. Some of this is cortical anticipation of the exercise that is to be done, but there may also be a reflex component stimulated by mechanical receptors in the leg muscles and tendons.

Voluntary control of breathing enables the breathing pattern to be altered in order to speak, eat, etc. These adjustments happen sub-consciously; but if they intrude into consciousness, they can result in dysfunctional breathing or hyperventilation.

Traditionally, involuntary stimulation of breathing is driven by hypoxia, hypercapnia, or acidosis. During the early part of a CPEX, however, ventilation increases steadily without any hint of hypoxia, hypercapnia, or acidosis. There must be other factors involved, for example, receptors which respond to change in airflow, intra-thoracic pressure, lung and chest-wall volume, or the degree of distension of pulmonary vessels.

Once the subject reaches the anaerobic threshold (AT), buffering of lactate by bicarbonate (HCO_3^-) keeps the pH normal for a while, but then acidaemia develops. The carotid bodies sense this change in pH and stimulate ventilation.

Further reading

Arena R, Guazzi M, Myers J. Prognostic value of end-tidal carbon dioxide during exercise testing in heart failure. Int J Cardiol. 2007 Apr 12;117(1):103–8. PubMed PMID: 16843545.

Cherniack NS, Longobardo GS. Cheyne-Stokes breathing. An instability in physiologic control. N Engl J Med. 1973 May 3;288(18):952–7. PubMed PMID: 4571351.

Diaz O, Villafranca C, Ghezzo H, Borzone G, Leiva A, Milic-Emili J, et al. Breathing pattern and gas exchange at peak exercise in COPD patients with and without tidal flow limitation at rest. Eur Respir J. 2001 Jun;17(6):1120–7. PubMed PMID: 11491153.

Holverda S, Bogaard HJ, Groepenhoff H, Postmus PE, Boonstra A, Vonk-Noordegraaf A. Cardiopulmonary exercise test characteristics in patients with chronic obstructive pulmonary disease and associated pulmonary hypertension. Respiration. 2008;76(2):160–7. PubMed PMID: 17960052.

Nemati S, Edwards BA, Sands SA, Berger PJ, Wellman A, Verghese GC, et al. Model-based characterization of ventilatory stability using spontaneous breathing. J Appl Physiol. 2011 Jul;111(1):55–67. PubMed PMID: 21474696. PubMed Central PMCID: 3137535.

Chapter 8

Respiratory exchange ratio

Key points

- The respiratory exchange ratio (RER) is the ratio of carbon dioxide output (VCO_2)/oxygen uptake (VO_2).
- Beyond the anaerobic threshold (AT), the RER increases above 1.0: VCO_2 rises more steeply, reflecting the production of carbon dioxide (CO_2) from the buffering of lactic acid, whereas VO_2—by definition—cannot increase.
- Subjects with dysfunctional breathing have erratic RER traces.

8.1 What is the RER?

It is time for another derived parameter: the RER is the VCO_2 divided by VO_2:

$$RER = VCO_2 \ / \ VO_2.$$

8.2 Why is RER measured?

The RER helps with a couple of things:

1. It gives a way of determining the AT.
2. It shows if the subject is hyperventilating.

8.3 What should the RER be?

If VCO_2 and VO_2 are both plotted against time during a cardiopulmonary exercise test (CPEX; Figure 8.1), VCO_2 is slightly less than VO_2 during the first part of the test, i.e. the RER (VCO_2/VO_2) is less than 1.0. At the end of the test, VCO_2 is greater than VO_2, so the RER will be greater than 1.0.

A plot of RER against time shows the same thing but is simpler than trying to see if the VO_2 line is above or below the VCO_2 line (Figure 8.2).

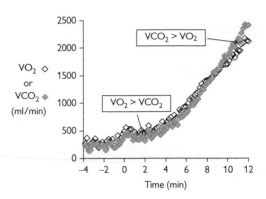

Fig. 8.1 Increase in VO_2 and VCO_2 during a CPEX.

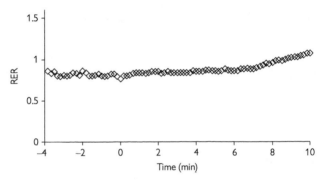

Fig. 8.2 Normal rise in RER during a CPEX.

Learning point

The RER (VCO_2/VO_2) should be less than 1.0 in the early part of a CPEX.

Physiology

RER

There are several reasons why the RER is less than 1.0. Firstly, the cells may produce slightly less CO_2 than the O_2 they consume, particularly if they are metabolising fat rather than glucose. (This is the respiratory quotient of the cells, which is sometimes confused with the RER of the whole person).

Secondly, some of the CO_2 dissolves in water and becomes part of the bicarbonate (HCO_3^-) buffering pool of the body. If some of the carbon in the CO_2 produced by the cells in muscle were labelled, some of it would ultimately show up as HCO_3^- excreted in the kidneys. There is no similar alternative for O_2.

The buffering capacity of the HCO_3^- system is much greater than that available for O_2, so any change in CO_2 has a much slower effect on the levels in the blood than is the case for O_2. These slower kinetics also make the RER a bit lower during a CPEX.

8.4 **RER and the AT**

Beyond the AT (see Chapter 9), the subject starts to exhale more CO_2 (produced from the buffering of lactic acid by HCO_3^-). At the AT, the two lines cross; at this point, VCO_2 and VO_2 are the same, so the RER must be 1.0. This is one way of determining the AT (the middle of the bottom row on a nine-panel display).

8.5 **Hyperventilation**

In Figure 8.3, the RER is a bit variable until the subject starts to exercise. This is not unusual, with a bit of hyperventilation until the subject relaxes.

Hyperventilation causes increased washout of CO_2 from the alveoli. On the other hand, increased ventilation cannot get any more O_2 into the body, because O_2 is poorly soluble and the haemoglobin (Hb) in red blood cells is already fully saturated. As a result, the RER is greater than 1.0.

In this context, hyperventilation is 'alveolar' hyperventilation: if lung disease has led to a very high dead space (Vd), hyperventilation may be necessary to get CO_2 out, but the RER will be normal. This topic will be discussed more in the chapter on ventilatory equivalents for CO_2 (VEqCO_2; Chapter 10).

47

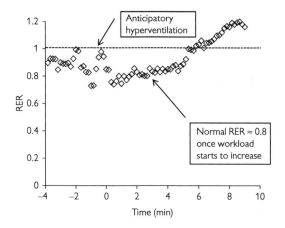

Fig. 8.3 Anticipatory hyperventilation during the initial phases of a CPEX, with a normal rise subsequently.

Clinical scenario

Dysfunctional breathing

A significant minority of patients that attend for exercise testing do so because of unexplained breathlessness.

Some of these patients will have abnormal ventilation unrelated to respiratory pathology: a circumstance that might be termed dysfunctional breathing, hyperventilation, or excessive anxiety. Indeed, some experts advocate the early use of a CPEX to definitively identify these individuals so they are not exposed to further, potentially hazardous, investigations and can begin to receive appropriate therapy.

CPEX is more specific than questionnaires for confirming hyperventilation; it can clearly demonstrate abnormal patterns such as frequent deep sighs and has the advantage of picking up occasional pathology, such as exercise-induced asthma.

Patients with dysfunctional breathing are less fit than the general population but usually reach somewhere around their predicted VO_2 max.

Respiratory rate will be disproportionately high throughout the exercise and recovery phases. Usually this is associated with a high overall ventilation, which washes out more CO_2 and causes the RER to be greater than 1.0 (Figure 8.4).

Tidal volume (Vt), however, may be lower than normal; so minute ventilation (VE) for a given exertion is not always elevated. Due to this elevated respiratory rate, ventilation is less efficient and ventilatory equivalents (VEq) are higher than would be expected (more of this later).

Subjects usually complain of greater respiratory symptoms than controls, but hyperventilation itself makes healthy individuals feel fatigued more rapidly.

Practical tip

An erratic RER during a CPEX is a pointer to the diagnosis of dysfunctional breathing.

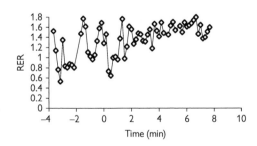

Fig. 8.4 High RER indicating hyperventilation or dysfunctional breathing.

Further reading

Cooper CB, Beaver WL, Cooper DM, Wasserman K. Factors affecting the components of the alveolar CO_2 output-O_2 uptake relationship during incremental exercise in man. Exp Physiol. 1992 Jan;77(1):51–64. PubMed PMID: 1543592.

Gardner WN, Meah MS, Bass C. Controlled study of respiratory responses during prolonged measurement in patients with chronic hyperventilation. Lancet. 1986 Oct 11;2(8511):826–30. PubMed PMID: 2876278.

Troosters T, Verstraete A, Ramon K, Schepers R, Gosselink R, Decramer M, et al. Physical performance of patients with numerous psychosomatic complaints suggestive of hyperventilation. Eur Respir J. 1999 Dec;14(6):1314–9. PubMed PMID: 10624760.

Chapter 9

Anaerobic threshold

Key points

- Beyond the anaerobic threshold (AT), anaerobic processes supplement aerobic metabolism, with production of lactic acid.
- Lactic acid is buffered by bicarbonate (HCO_3^-) to produce more carbon dioxide (CO_2).
- The AT should occur when the oxygen uptake (VO_2) is >40% of the predicted maximum oxygen uptake (VO_2max).
- A low AT is caused by impaired oxygen (O_2) delivery to muscles, usually because of heart disease or peripheral vascular disease.

9.1 What is the AT?

Over the years there has been much debate about the AT and what to call it. In this book it is assumed that, during an incremental exercise test, the AT is the point beyond which work is done by anaerobic as well as aerobic metabolism. It is important to remember that aerobic metabolism continues beyond the AT, but that it is supplemented by anaerobic processes. Although again there is considerable debate, for simplicity in this book it as assumed that anaerobic metabolism generates lactic acid in the muscles.

The AT referred to is that detected by analysis of exhaled gases, i.e. it is a 'respiratory' AT, rather than one determined by measurement of lactic acid in the blood or analysis of changes in the muscles themselves.

9.2 Why does the AT matter?

Whilst the scientists debate, athletes are well aware that there is a threshold below which the intensity of exercise can be sustained for fairly long periods, whereas above this threshold more intense exercise incurs a 'debt' which must be repaid.

As the external load increases progressively during a CPEX, as long as the subject is cycling at the correct speed, the work done gets steadily greater until they stop. Oxygen uptake (VO_2), however, tails off towards the peak of exercise. So how does the work done continue to increase? Well, aerobic metabolism must be supplemented by anaerobic processes (see Figure 9.1).

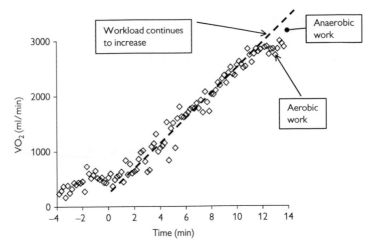

Fig. 9.1 Increase in work done during a cardiopulmonary exercise test (CPEX) continues to rise as the workload increases, whereas the VO_2 tails off. The energy for the continued increase in work comes from anaerobic metabolism.

Learning point

Aerobic metabolism continues beyond the AT, but is supplemented by anaerobic processes.

9.3 HCO_3^- buffering of lactic acid

Initially, the hydrogen ions (H^+) from the lactic acid produced in muscle is buffered by HCO_3^-, producing water (H_2O) and carbon dioxide (CO_2):

$$H^+ + HCO_3^- \rightarrow H_2O + CO_2$$

The water is easy to get rid of, but where does the CO_2 go? It is eliminated by increasing ventilation, of course.

As shown previously in Figure 8.1, when carbon dioxide output (VCO_2) and VO_2 are both plotted against time (top right in a nine-panel format), the VCO_2 crosses the VO_2 graph at the AT and continues to rise as VO_2 tails off towards its maximal value. At approximately 5 min after the start of the test in this example, the CO_2 crosses the VO_2 line. At this point, VO_2 and VCO_2 are approximately 1800 ml/min. This is the first method of detecting the AT. In Figure 8.2, the same data could be plotted as the respiratory exchange ratio (RER); and the AT can then be seen as the point at which the RER becomes greater than 1.0.

9.4 **The V-slope method of detecting the AT**

If VCO_2 is plotted against VO_2, there is an inflexion point at the AT beyond which the slope is steeper, as VCO_2 increases more than VO_2. This occurs when the VO_2 is around 1800 ml/min in this example. This is called the 'V-slope' method of determining the AT (right in the centre of a nine-panel display; see Figure 9.2).

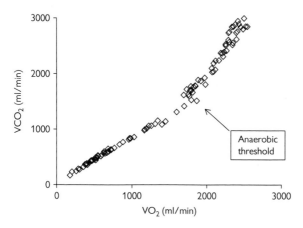

Fig. 9.2 V-slope plot: VO_2 plotted against VCO_2, with an inflexion point at the AT.

Quite often the slope of this plot takes a more gradual curve, rather than a sharp inflexion, and it's much more difficult to choose which exact point to call the AT. This shows that this is a gradual transition, with anaerobic processes beginning to supplement aerobic processes, rather than a sudden switch (see Figure 9.3).

Learning point

Beyond the AT, VCO_2 increases more steeply than VO_2.

9.5 **Uncertainty about the AT**

There is one more method of determining the AT, using ventilatory equivalents (Chapter 10). One of the problems of having several different methods is that they may not agree, so there can be some uncertainty about where to put the AT. Indeed, in some subjects it may be impossible to decide where to put it, particularly if the CPEX was very brief (Figure 9.4).

Practical tip

Always look at the graphical display to check which point has been chosen to call the AT.

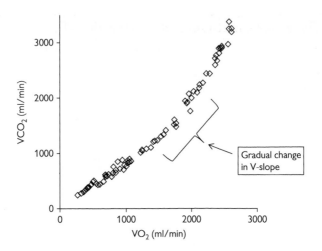

Fig. 9.3 V-slope plot, with a gradual inflexion as anaerobic metabolism slowly begins to produce a rise in VCO_2.

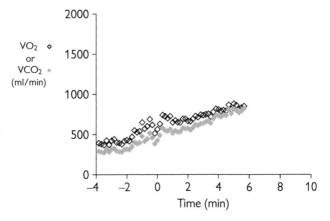

Fig. 9.4 VO_2 remaining greater than VCO_2 throughout the CPEX in a subject with lung disease, implying that the AT has not been reached.

9.6 **What is a normal AT?**

The AT should be greater than 40% of predicted maximum oxygen output (VO_2max). In trained athletes, this could be higher—even up to 80%.

The AT should be 40% or more of the **predicted** VO_2max, not the actual VO_2max.

9.7 **What causes a low AT?**

Anaerobic metabolism occurs when the circulation is not able to deliver enough oxygen (O_2) to meet the metabolic needs of the tissues. This may occur at lower than normal exercise intensity during a CPEX for three main reasons:

- The cardiac output is low.
- The blood vessels to the legs are obstructed.
- The peripheral oxygen saturation (SpO_2) of arterial blood is low.

So, the AT then gives us some additional information about how the body is performing during exercise, using the information in Table 9.1.

The unfit subject

As the population becomes more sedentary and medicine becomes more defensive, unfit individuals reporting exercise limitation are increasingly likely to end up on a CPEX test list. The amount of exercise a person could perform is related to their physical fitness and the severity and type of any disease they may have. So if a line is drawn to specify the 'normal' result for any single measurement of fitness, unfit individuals may well fall below this and fit people with mild disease may not. What are the changes that occur with exercise or lack of it, and how do they impact on CPEX findings?

The effects of exercise are wide-ranging, complex, and not all well understood even if they are reproducibly demonstrable. Exercise (especially if >80% of maximum heart rate (HR)) results in muscle and endothelial shear stress, stretch strain, and local hypoxia. This leads to an increase in signalling molecules which affect both acute and chronic changes in the transcription of genes involved in angiogenesis, mitochondrial oxidative capacity, and cellular survival, amongst others. Exercise also alters energy balance and so clearly modulates the potential adverse endocrine effects of obesity such as those driven by hyperleptinaemia.

Although hypertrophy is common to all exercised muscles, it is the increase in cardiac muscle and resultant cardiac output that has the greatest influence on exercise capacity. Increased cardiac output also means that a lower resting HR can maintain a perfusing blood pressure and that increases in blood pressure can be attained when necessary with less emphasis on increased systemic resistance. Fitness is also increased by improving microvascular O_2 extraction in the muscles through increased capillarity. This is a result of both the enlargement of existing vessels and the formation of new ones; and this increased efficiency results in the need for a lower resting minute ventilation (VE). As mitochondrial oxidative capacity increases, lipid handling is also beneficially altered (more high-density lipoprotein (HDL), less low-density lipoprotein (LDL)) and the reduction in lipid deposition (amongst other factors) improves insulin resistance. The effect of exercise on the vascular endothelium also results in the release of factors which lead to a slowing in the age-related decline in vasodilatative ability and a reduction in fibrinogen and platelet adhesiveness.

	AT (% predicted VO$_2$max)
Table 9.1 AT in different clinical states.	
Trained athlete	61–80
Normal	51–60
Deconditioned/mild disease	40–50
Abnormal	<40

Further reading

Astrand P-O, Rodahl K. Textbook of Work Physiology, 3rd edition (1986) London: McGraw-Hill.

Beaver WL, Wasserman K, Whipp BJ. Bicarbonate buffering of lactic acid generated during exercise. J Appl Physiol. 1986 Feb;60(2):472–8. PubMed PMID: 3949651.

Hopker JG, Jobson SA, Pandit JJ. Controversies in the physiological basis of the 'anaerobic threshold' and their implications for clinical cardiopulmonary exercise testing. Anaesthesia. 2011 Feb;66(2):111–23. PubMed PMID: 21254986.

Chapter 10

Ventilatory equivalents

Key points

- The ventilatory equivalents for oxygen ($VEqO_2$) are the amounts of ventilation (ml/min) divided by how much oxygen (O_2) is taken in (ml/min).
- $VEqO_2$ fall during the initial part of a cardiopulmonary exercise test (CPEX), as ventilation and perfusion become more even throughout the lungs.
- Beyond the anaerobic threshold (AT), $VEqO_2$ rise as ventilation increases (stimulated by carbon dioxide output (VCO_2)) without any increase in oxygen uptake (VO_2).

10.1 What are ventilatory equivalents?

The final 'derived' parameter in this book is the ventilatory equivalent. The $VEqO_2$ is simply the minute ventilation (VE) divided by the amount of O_2 taken up. In other words, how many millilitres of air went in and out of the lungs to get a millilitre of O_2 in. It can be thought of as an index of how well the lungs work—lots of air in and out without much O_2 taken up by the body sounds bad.

Ventilatory equivalents (VEq) are one of those odd things that have no units: VE is in ml/min, and so is VO_2; ml/min divided by ml/min leaves nothing—hence a unit-less index.

10.2 Why do VEq matter?

In the first part of a CPEX, the $VEqO_2$ may gradually fall (Figure 10.1). The lowest point of the VEq is where the lungs are working at their best. How many millilitres of ventilation per millilitre of O_2 taken in at this nadir gives some idea of how good the lungs are.

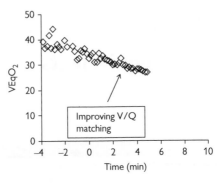

Fig. 10.1 $VEqO_2$ fall as cardiac output increases and ventilation (V)/perfusion (Q) matching becomes more even.

Physiology

Ventilation-perfusion matching

At rest, in the upright posture, there is a small gradient in ventilation (V) from the top to the bottom of the lungs. There is a much more pronounced gradient in lung perfusion (Q), with lots of blood passing through distended blood vessels in the lung base, whilst at the apex the vessels have little or no blood in them.

During exercise, cardiac output increases and blood vessels towards the apex of the lungs are recruited (Figure 10.2). Perfusion of the lungs becomes more uniform, and as a result, there is better matching of V and Q.

10.3 **Why do $VEqO_2$ rise beyond the AT?**

In the later stages of a CPEX (past the AT), the $VEqO_2$ rise. At first glance, it might appear as if the lungs were becoming less effective at taking O_2 into the body, but this is not the case. Beyond the AT, ventilation increases to blow off the carbon dioxide (CO_2) generated by buffering lactic acid. The VO_2 can't increase any further, because the blood flowing out of the lungs is already fully saturated (which is why anaerobic metabolism has kicked in). Hence the amount of ventilation per millilitre of O_2—the 'ventilatory equivalent' for O_2—starts to increase suddenly. It looks as if the lungs are less efficient at getting O_2 in, but actually the main reason for this increase is the need to get more CO_2 out (Figure 10.3—this is usually the right-hand graph in the middle row of a nine-panel display). We now have four ways of looking for the AT (Box 10.1).

Box 10.1 Four ways of looking for the AT

1. On a plot of VCO_2 and VO_2 against time, the VCO_2 starts to increase faster and crosses the VO_2 line.
2. When VCO_2 is plotted against VO_2, the slope changes to become steeper.
3. The respiratory exchange ratio (RER) increases to a value greater than 1.0.
4. The $VEqO_2$ suddenly start to increase.

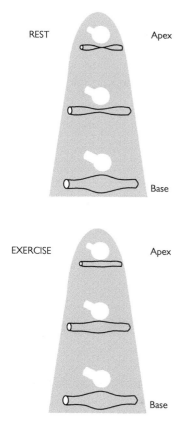

Fig. 10.2 Blood flow (Q) through vessels (with black lines) and ventilation (V) of alveoli (white spaces) in different regions of the lung. Q becomes more even on exercise, which improves V-Q matching. The gradient for V is much less marked than for Q.

10.4 **End-tidal O$_2$ concentration**

Some CPEX equipment will display end-tidal concentrations of O$_2$ and CO$_2$. The idea is that the gas exhaled right at the end of expiration has come from deep within the lungs, i.e. from the alveoli. (This will be a mixture of gas from all alveoli, some of them well perfused and some under-perfused.)

During the early part of a CPEX, more and more O$_2$ is taken up from the alveoli into the blood, as V-Q matching improves. As a result, there is less O$_2$ in the expired gas. In other words, the end-tidal O$_2$ falls (Figure 10.4).

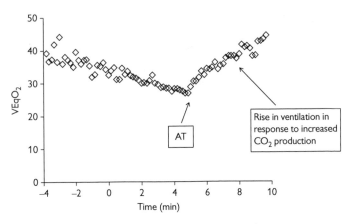

Fig. 10.3 VEqO$_2$ rise beyond the AT, when VO$_2$ leads to an increase in ventilation.

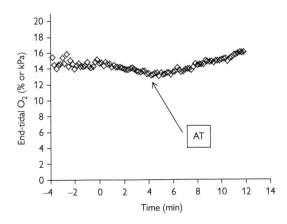

Fig. 10.4 End-tidal O$_2$ levels fall as more O$_2$ is taken out of the inspired air but rise again once V increases past the AT.

Past the AT, however, ventilation increases without any more O$_2$ being taken up by the blood. As a result, the expired gas starts to look more like inspired air, so the end-tidal level rises again, back towards that of inspired air.

10.5 **VEq for CO$_2$**

The VEq for CO$_2$ (VEqCO$_2$) are calculated in a similar way to those for O$_2$: how many millilitres of V are needed to get 1 ml of CO$_2$ out. They will be used in the next chapter to look at the respiratory compensation point (RCP).

Further reading

Kinnula VL, Sovijarvi AR. Elevated ventilatory equivalents during exercise in patients with hyperventilation syndrome. Respiration. 1993;60(5):273–8. PubMed PMID: 8284522.

O'Donnell DE, D'Arsigny C, Fitzpatrick M, Webb KA. Exercise hypercapnia in advanced chronic obstructive pulmonary disease: the role of lung hyperinflation. Am J Respir Crit Care Med. 2002 Sep 1;166(5):663–8. PubMed PMID: 12204862.

Whipp BJ, Wasserman K. Alveolar-arterial gas tension differences during graded exercise. J Appl Physiol. 1969 Sep;27(3):361–5. PubMed PMID: 5804133.

Further reading

Chapter 11

Respiratory compensation point

> ### Key points
> - The respiratory compensation point (RCP) is seen when acidaemia takes over from carbon dioxide (CO_2) as the stimulus for ventilation.
> - The presence of a clear RCP implies a pretty maximal effort by the subject.

11.1 What are the ventilatory equivalents for CO_2?

The ventilatory equivalents for CO_2 ($VEqCO_2$) is the number of millilitres of minute ventilation (VE) for each millilitre of CO_2 exhaled. It improves early on in a cardio-pulmonary exercise test (CPEX), implying that there is less ventilation of dead space volume (Vd), as blood starts to flow through alveolar units that were previously unperfused and hence acting as dead space.

11.2 The RCP

As with the ventilatory equivalents for oxygen ($VEqO_2$) plot, the slope of the plot of $VEqCO_2$ against time increases towards the end of exercise. The point at which the slope changes is a bit later than the anaerobic threshold (AT). It is called the RCP and is shown in Figure 11.1. It isn't always there, and it doesn't always happen much later than the AT. Nevertheless, if it is there, it shows that the subject tried pretty hard during the test and became acidaemic.

> ### Learning point
> *The presence of a clear RCP implies the development of sufficient lactic acid to produce acidaemia.*

As with end-tidal oxygen (O_2) concentrations, increasing ventilation leads the CO_2 values to become closer to those of inspired air (Figure 11.2).

In patients with lung disease, they may not be able to exercise to the point where they become acidaemic. Even if they do, if ventilation is limiting exercise capacity, then there would be no possibility of increasing ventilation to compensate for acidosis, so we wouldn't see a change in the slope of the VE/VCO_2 graph (i.e. there

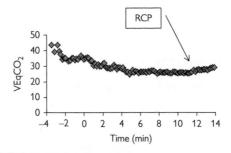

Fig. 11.1 Increase in $VEqCO_2$ beyond the RCP.

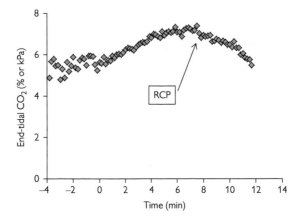

Fig. 11.2 End-tidal CO_2 falls past the RCP, when acidaemia begins to stimulate ventilation.

is no RCP). Conversely, the presence of an RCP implies that ventilation was not limiting exercise.

Practical tip
If there is a clear RCP, significant lung disease is unlikely.

When the $VEqO_2$ and $VEqCO_2$ are plotted on the same graph, the AT can be seen on the O_2 plot, with the RCP occurring slightly later on the CO_2 plot. The part between these two points is where muscle acidosis is effectively buffered by bicarbonate (HCO_3^-), preventing acidaemia but generating CO_2 (Figure 11.3).

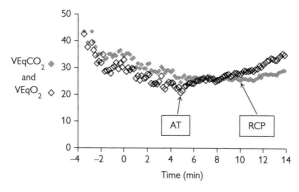

Fig. 11.3 $VEqO_2$ and $VEqCO_2$, showing the presence of an AT and an RCP.

Practical tip

The nadir on the CO_2 plot is often much less clear cut than for O_2—more of a curve than a sharp angle.

Clinical scenario

Sub-maximal effort

When looking at CPEX results, it is quite important to decide how far the subject pushed themselves. Observing the patient gives a good indication of how hard they tried, but subjects who have made a maximal effort will also show some if not all of the following:
- *a high maximum heat rate (HR)*
- *a flattening of the oxygen intake (VO_2) at peak exercise, implying that they are approaching maximal VO_2*
- *a clear RCP.*

11.3 **Efficiency of ventilation**

The lowest point or nadir on the $VEqCO_2$ plot indicates the point at which the lungs are at their most efficient in terms of eliminating CO_2. If the $VEqCO_2$ are more than 30, this implies that there is a high Vd/tidal volume (Vt) ratio. (Calculation of Vd/Vt requires measurement of the arterial CO_2, but many CPEX systems will try to estimate this from the end-tidal CO_2).

If the mechanics of the lungs are abnormal, the subject won't be able to achieve very high ventilation; so by the time the subjects stops exercising, $VEqCO_2$ may not be particularly high. The ability to increase ventilation easily, but with poor gas exchange, is characteristic of pulmonary vascular disease (Figure 11.4).

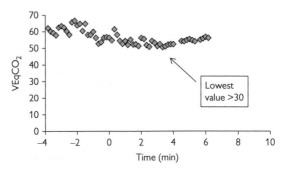

Fig. 11.4 High VEqCO$_2$ implying inefficiency of the lungs in terms of alveolar ventilation, for example in pulmonary vascular disease.

Learning point

If the VEqCO$_2$ do not fall below 30, this implies that there is something wrong with gas exchange in the lungs (with a high Vd/Vt ratio). Most commonly, this is pulmonary vascular disease.

11.4 **Dysfunctional breathing**

If the subject is anxious and hyperventilating, ventilation will be high. As a result, the arterial CO$_2$ partial pressure (PaCO$_2$) falls, and the 'driving pressure' to get CO$_2$ from the blood into the alveoli is therefore less. This combination of high ventilation and low CO$_2$ output is the same as we see if the lungs are diseased, with a high Vd/Vt ratio.

Clearly differentiating lung disease from dysfunctional breathing is really important. The clue is usually the irregularity of ventilation: subjects with dysfunctional breathing have a much more irregular ventilatory pattern, which will be seen on the plots of time vs VE, respiratory exchange ratio (RER), and VEqCO$_2$.(Figure 11.5).

Practical tip

Look for irregularity in VE, RER, and VEqCO$_2$ in order to distinguish dysfunctional breathing from lung disease.

11.5 **VEqCO$_2$ and prognosis**

As mentioned previously, a high VE/VCO$_2$ (i.e. a high Vd/Vt) indicates a poor prognosis in a patient with heart failure. Using VEqCO$_2$ to quantify severity (Table 11.1) can be used in preoperative exercise testing (Chapter 16).

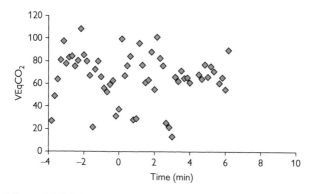

Fig. 11.5 Highly variable $VEqCO_2$ in a subject with dysfunctional breathing and hyperventilation.

Table 11.1 Maximum oxygen uptake (VO_2max) and $VEqCO_2$ as indicators for the severity of cardiorespiratory impairment.

Severity	VO_2max (ml kg/min)	$VEqCO_2$
Normal	>20	<30
Mild	16–20	30–35
Moderate	10–15	36–45
Severe	<10	>45

Further reading

Maughan R, Gleeson M, Greenhaff P. Biochemistry of Exercise and Training (1997) New York: Oxford University Press.

Meyer T, Faude O, Scharhag J, Urhausen A, Kindermann W. Is lactic acidosis a cause of exercise induced hyperventilation at the respiratory compensation point? Br J Sports Med. 2004 Oct;38(5):622–5. PubMed PMID: 15388552. Pubmed Central PMCID: 1724908.

Chapter 12

Oxygen saturation

> **Key points**
> - A fall in peripheral oxygen saturation (SpO$_2$) of more than 4% is unusual during a cardiopulmonary exercise test (CPEX).
> - Disorders of the lung and pulmonary circulation are the commonest causes of oxygen (O$_2$) desaturation.
> - Patients with heart disease tend not to desaturate on exercise.
> - Atrial septal defects are common and may only open up to cause a right-to-left shunt when right heart pressures rise during a CPEX.

SpO$_2$ falls in patients with severe lung disease when they start to do even minimal exercise. Clearly this will happen if they are assessed using a CPEX. In the absence of lung disease, a fall in SpO$_2$ during the test is pretty unusual and indicates a significant problem with gas exchange. (If using a finger probe, check that the fall is not an artefact caused by the subject gripping the handlebars too tightly). At the end of a running race, everyone tends to be bright red, irrespective of how fit they are.

12.1 What is a fall in SpO$_2$?

A significant fall in SpO$_2$ is more than 4% from the resting value (Figure 12.1). This is usually shown on the bottom right-hand graph of a nine-panel display.). There are three main physiological reasons for O$_2$ desaturation on exercise (Box 12.1).

12.2 V-Q imbalance

At rest in the upright posture, more blood goes to the bottom of the lungs than the top. When cardiac output increases on exercise, blood flow becomes more even as the pulmonary vessels towards the top of the lung open up. In other words, V-Q matching becomes more even.

What happens if the lungs are diseased? In a patient with chronic obstructive pulmonary disease (COPD), some areas of the lungs will be over-inflated. In these areas, the pulmonary vascular tree is stretched very thinly, and there isn't much capacity to accommodate more blood when the cardiac output increases on exercise. The blood has to go to other parts of the lung, which become over-perfused. The result is hypoxaemia.

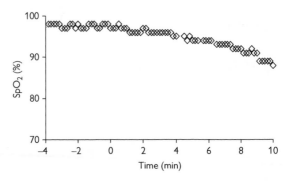

Fig. 12.1 Falling SpO$_2$ during a CPEX.

Box 12.1 Causes of O$_2$ desaturation during a CPEX

- Impaired diffusion
- Ventilation (V)-perfusion(Q) imbalance
- Right-to-left cardiac shunt
- Artefactual (poor signal from the probe)

Learning point

A fall in SpO$_2$ of >4% during a CPEX is abnormal and implies the presence of lung disease, pulmonary vascular disease, or the opening of a right-to-left shunt.

Physiology

Impaired diffusion

When blood enters the lung, the oxygen partial pressure (PO$_2$) is approximately 5 kPa. It pretty rapidly increases to reach a value which is close to, but just below, the PO$_2$ in the alveoli (Figure 12.2). (The difference between the alveolar and arterial PO$_2$ is referred to as the A-a gradient.)

During exercise, cardiac output increases, and the blood flows more rapidly through the pulmonary capillaries. Nevertheless, there is still plenty of time for the blood to become fully saturated with haemoglobin (Hb). Oxygen desaturation does not occur on exercise if the lungs are normal (unless there is an intra-cardiac shunt). At the end of a running race, everyone is bright red, not blue.

If there is a problem with diffusion, perhaps because the alveolar walls are thickened by inflammation or fibrosis, it takes longer for the PO$_2$ of the blood in all the pulmonary capillaries to reach the same level (just below the alveolar value; Figure 12.3). Any reduction in the time the blood spends in the capillaries when the subject starts to exercise will result in a fall in arterial PO$_2$ and hence SpO$_2$.

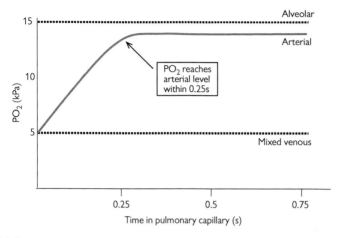

Fig. 12.2 The normal rise in PO_2 in the blood, from mixed venous to arterial levels within 0.25 s of entering the pulmonary capillaries.

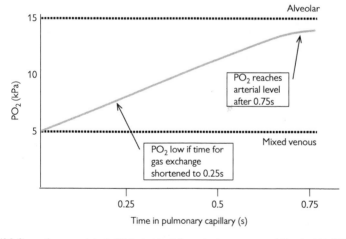

Fig. 12.3 Slower than normal rise in PO_2 in the blood, from mixed venous to arterial levels within 0.75 s of entering the pulmonary capillaries.

Learning point

A CPEX is an excellent way of stressing the gas exchange capabilities of the lungs and unmasking diffusion limitation which may not have been apparent on tests done with the patient at rest.

12.3 **Atrial septal defects**

A patient with a significant right-to-left shunt will probably be cyanosed at rest, and the problem will have been detected clinically or on tests prior to a CPEX. However, it is worth mentioning small atrial septal defects, which only open up on exercise when the pressure in the right heart rises. This will cause a sudden fall in SpO_2. As many as 20% of the population have a patent foramen ovale.

Learning point

Atrial septal defects are common and may only open up on exercise.

If the lungs aren't working well, or blood is passing through an intra-cardiac shunt and bypassing the lungs, then the exhaled air will start to look more like inhaled air, i.e. not much will have happened to it whilst it was in the lungs. This can be seen on the end-tidal gas concentration plots.

12.4 **O_2 desaturation and O_2 pulse**

One final point to note about subjects who desaturate: if not very much O_2 is taken up by the blood passing through the lungs, but the heart rate (HR) continues to rise, then inevitably there will be a fall in the O_2 pulse.

Practical tip

If the O_2 pulse doesn't rise normally during a CPEX, check the SpO_2 trace just in case this is caused by failure to oxygenate the blood up to normal arterial levels.

Further reading

Badesch DB, Abman SH, Simonneau G, Rubin LJ, McLaughlin VV. Medical therapy for pulmonary arterial hypertension: updated ACCP evidence-based clinical practice guidelines. Chest. 2007 Jun;131(6):1917–28. PubMed PMID: 17565025.

Deboeck G, Niset G, Lamotte M, Vachiery JL, Naeije R. Exercise testing in pulmonary arterial hypertension and in chronic heart failure. Eur Respir J. 2004 May;23(5):747–51. PubMed PMID: 15176691.

King TE, Jr, Tooze JA, Schwarz MI, Brown KR, Cherniack RM. Predicting survival in idiopathic pulmonary fibrosis: scoring system and survival model. Am J Respir Crit Care Med. 2001 Oct 1;164(7):1171–81. PubMed PMID: 11673205.

Mak VH, Bugler JR, Roberts CM, Spiro SG. Effect of arterial oxygen desaturation on six minute walk distance, perceived effort, and perceived breathlessness in patients with airflow limitation. Thorax. 1993 Jan;48(1):33–8. PubMed PMID: 8434350. Pubmed Central PMCID: 464235.

Part 3

Using cardiopulmonary exercise test data

Chapter 13

Presentation of results

13.1 Tables

CPEX reports too often have pages full of numbers. There are a small number of key parameters, all of which have already been covered, which are needed in order to decide what is wrong.

For oxygen uptake (VO_2), heart rate (HR), and minute ventilation (VE), the maximum recorded value should be compared with the predicted value to see if it reaches 80% (Table 13.1).

With AT, the observed value needs to be compared with the predicted maximum oxygen uptake (VO_2max), which is a bit more cumbersome to present in a table (Table 13.2).

There are lots of other parameters which could put in a table, but a graph is often more informative.

13.2 Graphs

Graphs show what happened during the course of the test. The first thing to do is to look at the VO_2, HR, and VE traces to check how the subject progressed up to the maximum value presented in the table. (In most nine-panel displays, these graphs are the first three across the top row.) A low maximum minute ventilation (VEmax), for example, has different implications if there had been a steady rise in ventilation during the test, as opposed to the erratic pattern of dysfunctional breathing.

After looking at VE, check the HR graph. It makes sense to look at the O_2 pulse at the same time, as it is usually on the same plot.

Then look at VO_2 and the carbon dioxide output (VCO_2), noting how they rise and if they cross. This gives the first estimate of the anaerobic threshold (AT).

Table 13.1 Maximum values of oxygen uptake (VO_2), heart rate (HR), and minute ventilation (VE) in a subject undergoing a cardiopulmonary exercise test.

Peak exercise:

	Measured	% predicted
VO_2 (ml/min)	2006	92
HR (bpm)	178	90
VE (l/min)	59	63

Table 13.2 Cardiopulmonary exercise test data at peak exercise and the anaerobic threshold (AT).

	Peak exercise		AT	
	Measured	% predicted	Measured	% predicted VO_2max
VO_2 (ml/min)	2006	92	1205	55
HR (bpm)	178	90		
VE (l/min)	59	63		

Practical tip

When learning to look at an electrocardiogram (ECG), leads are looked at in a fairly systematic order: I, II, III, aVR, aVL, aVF, and then the V leads. A similar approach should be adopted when starting to look at CPEX graphs, looking first along Graphs 1, 2, and 3 from left to right on the top row. Then on to 4, 5, and 6 from left to right on the middle row, finishing off with 7, 8, and 9 on the bottom row.

The middle row of a nine-panel display will usually have VE/VCO_2, where it can be noted if VE is too high and if there is a compensation point. The middle graph is the V-slope plot, showing the AT. The graph at the far end of the middle row, ventilatory equivalents (VEq), shows the AT and RCP again and indicates whether there was a problem with gas exchange.

Along the bottom row, tidal volume (Vt)/VE can identify dysfunctional breathing or lung disease. In the middle, the respiratory exchange ratio (RER) helps with the AT and dysfunctional breathing again. The bottom right plot gives us peripheral oxygen saturation (SpO_2) and, if they are available, end-tidal oxygen (O_2) and carbon dioxide (CO_2).

Having started with a pretty methodical approach, look back at the other graphs, just to check that everything fits with the conclusions drawn from the first impression. For example, a high RER throughout the CPEX in Graph 8 might prompt a second look at VE (Graphs 1 and 4), VEq (Graph 6), and Vt/VE (Graph 7). In fact, the nine-panel display is designed to make this sort of approach easier.

Practical tip

Don't over-interpret the graphs of a CPEX if the VO₂max is normal: significant pathology is unlikely.

13.3 **Ventilation, circulation, and gas exchange**

An alternative format presents groups of graphs that allow the assessment of the circulatory, ventilatory, and gas exchange responses to exercise separately. For circulation, heart rate (HR), VO_2, and O_2 pulse are plotted against time (or VO_2 against HR instead of O_2 pulse). For ventilation, VE is plotted against time, and VE/VCO_2, Vt/ VE, and VEq are plotted against time. For gas exchange, AT (from V-slope, RER, and VEq) is plotted against SpO_2. The printed tables generated by the CPEX equipment may subdivide the summary data along these lines, often with several other derived parameters as well.

Practical tip

CPEX results are presented in lots of different ways. Looking through the data and graphs systematically allows the brain to learn where to find the information that it wants. At first, it may help to use a highlighter pen on a paper copy of the results, circling key points on the graphs or tables and drawing lines between them.

13.4 **Algorithms**

Decisions about what is going on during a CPEX can be made by looking at what happens to a few key parameters. An initial hypothesis may then be modified or confirmed after reviewing other parameters. This sort of thought process can be synthesized into an algorithm. For the first few decisions, an algorithm might look something like Figure 13.1.

As more complicated parameters are added, then more complex algorithms with subsidiary branching points are needed. A different version will also be needed to make allowance for the possibility that the AT may not be identified reliably. This approach is considered in much more detail by Wasserman et al (see Reference Texts).

13.5 **Automated analysis**

Interpreting CPEX results is a pretty sophisticated skill. Computers are not yet advanced enough to produce particularly helpful interpretations of the results.

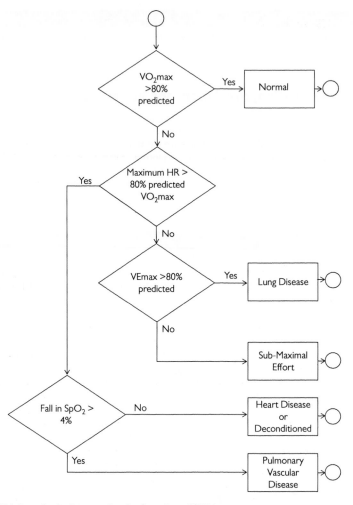

Fig. 13.1 Example of a diagnostic algorithm for analysing CPEX data.

Further reading

American Thoracic Society, American College of Chest Physicians. ATS/ACCP Statement on cardiopulmonary exercise testing. Am J Respir Crit Care Med. 2003 Jan 15;167(2):211–77. PubMed PMID: 12524257.

Guazzi M, Adams V, Conraads V, Halle M, Mezzani A, Vanhees L, et al. Clinical recommendations for cardiopulmonary exercise testing data assessment in specific patient populations. Eur Heart J. 2012 Dec;33(23):2917–27. PubMed PMID: 22952138.

Chapter 14

Exercise prescription

Key points

- Exercise works best if undertaken daily.
- It should be at least moderate in intensity, getting the heart rate (HR) above 75% of the predicted maximum.
- Start slowly and build up.

14.1 **Exercise as therapy**

If there were a cheap drug that reduced all-cause mortality in a dose dependent fashion, it would be widely known how to prescribe it. Medical professionals tend not to be quite so conversant with exercise prescription, despite it having this effect. The health benefits are not only through a reduction in cardiovascular risk factors and type 2 diabetes, but also through increased independence and reduced risk of falling in older people and a robust association with reduced incidence of common cancers such as breast and colon.

General recommendations for exercise are in broad agreement that individuals should aim for 30 min of moderate exercise on most days or 20 min vigorous exercise thrice weekly (or combinations thereof). Further benefits come from weight-bearing exercise and activities that improve other components of fitness such as muscular strength, flexibility, or agility. All periods of exercise should also have additional warm-up and cool-down periods. Clearly, the definitions of moderate and vigorous exercise we choose are important, and Table 14.1 gives a few examples of such activities.

Bear in mind that, having subjected the individual to an exercise test, a more individualized HR range can be chosen for each exercise category (from the plot of HR against oxygen uptake (VO_2)) if the patient wishes to use a HR monitor. If they opt for a pedometer, half an hour's brisk walking equates to around 3500 steps, and 10000 steps per day is an overall target in the physically active.

14.2 **Exercise advice after a cardiopulmonary exercise test**

It is most likely exercise advice will be given as general encouragement rather than a precise prescription, leaving this didactic approach for experts in the area and more

Table 14.1 Intensity of exercise related to percentage of maximum heart rate (%HRmax) and percentage of maximum oxygen uptake (%VO$_2$max), with examples.

		Light	Moderate	Vigorous
%VO$_2$max		20–40	40–60	>60
%HRmax		50–65	65–75	>75
Example activities	**Walking**	Walking whilst shopping	Walking briskly	Jogging
	Chores	Washing up	Washing the car	Digging
	Recreation	Playing instrument	Ballroom dancing	Cycling uphill
	Sport	Fishing	Golf (no buggy)	Basketball game

serious athletes. A similar approach should be tried as for smoking cessation or weight loss when supporting and motivating patients in relation to exercise: assess the patient's fears and readiness for change, advise on the potential benefits in a personalized manner and improve their knowledge, give options for change, and provide support and follow-up.

As would be expected, getting sedentary people to exercise can be as difficult as stopping someone from smoking; but any amount of activity is of benefit in this group. Keeping people exercising usually depends on finding a range of activities the patient enjoys and building up activity over months, taking care to increase only intensity or frequency, or duration of exercise at any stage to minimise injury risk. This slow build-up from a low level is particularly important in older individuals, and involvement of physiotherapy colleagues should be considered to ensure muscle strengthening (e.g. stair climbing) and balance exercises (e.g. heel stands, tandem walking) are included for this group.

Further reading

Casaburi R. Principles of exercise training. Chest. 1992 May;101(5 Suppl):263S–7S. PubMed PMID: 1576847.

Gulati M, Black HR, Shaw LJ, Arnsdorf MF, Merz CN, Lauer MS, et al. The prognostic value of a nomogram for exercise capacity in women. N Engl J Med. 2005 Aug 4;353(5):468–75. PubMed PMID: 16079370.

Laukkanen JA, Rauramaa R, Salonen JT, Kurl S. The predictive value of cardiorespiratory fitness combined with coronary risk evaluation and the risk of cardiovascular and all-cause death. Intern Med. 2007 Aug;262(2):263–72. PubMed PMID: 17645594.

Mora S, Redberg RF, Cui Y, Whiteman MK, Flaws JA, Sharrett AR, et al. Ability of exercise testing to predict cardiovascular and all-cause death in asymptomatic women: a 20-year follow-up of the lipid research clinics prevalence study. JAMA. 2003 Sep 24;290(12):1600–7. PubMed PMID: 14506119.

Chapter 15

Clinical scenarios

Key points

- Characteristic cardiopulmonary exercise test (CPEX) patterns are described for several diseases.
- Few patients display all these characteristics.

Having worked through a number of different CPEX parameters, and along the way taken note of how they might be affected by certain clinical conditions, in this chapter the opposite approach is taken: the focus is on the clinical conditions themselves and how CPEX parameters are affected by them.

15.1 Heart disease

In patients with heart disease, cardiac output is likely to be low. This limits exercise capacity because of the inability of the circulation to transport sufficient oxygen (O_2) from the lungs to the muscles. The muscles must therefore start to use anaerobic processes earlier than normal.

At least some of the following should be seen:

- low maximum O_2 uptake (VO_2max)
- rapid early rise in heart rate (HR)
- low HR reserve
- O_2 pulse plateau, with peak value <10 ml/beat
- low anaerobic threshold (AT)
- high minute ventilation (VE)/carbon dioxide (CO_2) with ventilatory equivalents for CO_2 ($VEqCO_2$) >30 (because of high dead space volume (Vd)/tidal volume (Vt)).

As noted in the chapter on HR, 'chronotrophic insufficiency' can lead to impairment of exercise capacity, because HR fails to rise normally. Look out for this pattern in patients with heart disease.

Patients with heart failure sometimes have a rather 'noisy' VE, VO_2, or O_2-pulse plot. On closer inspection, a cyclical pattern may be seen which is the equivalent of Cheyne-Stokes respiration (Figure 15.1). This could represent 'under-damping' of respiratory control, caused by a low cardiac output with a delay in the respiratory control

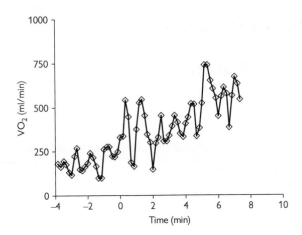

Fig. 15.1 Cyclical VO_2 in a patient with heart failure.

processes detecting a rise or fall in arterial carbon dioxide partial pressure ($PaCO_2$), or 'hunting' around a low $PaCO_2$, which is too near the apnoeic threshold.

Finally, look out for opening of a patent foramen ovale, when the development of a right-to-left shunt would lead to a fall in peripheral oxygen saturation (SpO_2), as well as the O_2 pulse. A compensatory increase in VE might occur, but since some blood would now bypass the lungs, the end-tidal gas would start to look more like inspired air.

15.2 **Lung disease**

Patients with lung problems tend to have problems with eliminating CO_2 rather than with delivering O_2 to the muscles (although the latter process does become important if the muscles start to desaturate). They should show at least some of the following during a CPEX:

- low VO_2max
- high HR reserve
- low VE reserve
- flat Vt/VE plot
- high $VEqCO_2$
- desaturation.

These patients are often unfit, so the AT may be low. However, it is not uncommon for them not to be able to get to the AT. It is also uncommon to see a clear respiratory compensation point (RCP), as they have usually stopped short of this point because of breathlessness.

15.3 **Pulmonary vascular disease**

Many patients with 'lung' disease actually have disruption of the pulmonary vasculature. Since the mechanics of breathing are fairly normal, these patients can increase their ventilation quite well, but they desaturate quickly. There is a low cardiac output because of obstruction of the pulmonary vascular tree. As a result, a CPEX will show:

- low VO_2max
- low HR reserve
- low O_2 pulse
- low AT
- high $VEqCO_2$
- desaturation.

15.4 **Peripheral vascular disease**

When peripheral vascular disease prevents O_2 from being delivered to the leg muscles, anaerobic metabolism kicks in far earlier than expected. As lactic acid builds up in the muscles, the subject develops pain and has to stop. On a CPEX there will be:

- low VO_2max
- high HR reserve
- high VE reserve
- low AT.

15.5 **Sub-maximal effort**

A sub-maximal effort could be due to volitional or motivational factors, but it also could be due to something like arthritic pain (in which case the 'sub-maximal' bit refers only to the cardiorespiratory aspects of the test).

Careful questioning of the patient as to what stopped them is clearly going to be key. A CPEX will show:

- low VO_2max
- high HR reserve
- high VE reserve
- normal AT
- no RCP.

15.6 **Muscle diseases**

Some muscle diseases cause characteristic patterns which resemble a sub-maximal effort, except that the AT is low. If VO_2max is low and the AT normal (or indeterminate), limb muscle pathology is unlikely, unless there are some pointers to muscle disease in the history or on clinical examination.

15.7 **Dysfunctional breathing**

A CPEX is a useful test when a patient complains of breathlessness but there is nothing wrong clinically or on initial investigation. Clues that suggest dysfunctional breathing as a diagnosis are:

- low VO_2max
- normal AT
- no RCP
- high VE at rest, with erratic rise on exercise
- high respiratory exchange ratio (RER) at rest with erratic rise on exercise
- erratic VEqCO$_2$.

Some of the patients coming up for a CPEX will have limited exercise tolerance or intrusive symptoms on exertion but may not have an underlying pathology to explain this. Their symptoms are often a result of excessive awareness of the normal sensations during exercise rather than a clear attempt to falsify illness, and many are reassured by the results of CPEX that there is nothing seriously amiss. To identify the patients displaying sub-maximal effort, look first at the peak values during the test and compare these to the predicted values: all will be lower than predicted, suggesting neither ventilatory nor cardiovascular limitation has occurred. Next, look for the AT. If it has been reached, there will usually be relatively little exercise time after it occurs (often less than 20% of total exercise time). If there is an inflection in the graph of carbon dioxide output (VCO_2) vs ventilation, this suggests that acidaemia is directly driving respiration and that the subject has produced maximal effort.

15.8 **Lack of fitness**

If a subject is unfit, or 'deconditioned', expect to see:

- low VO_2max
- low HR reserve
- high VE reserve
- maximum O_2 pulse <15 ml/beat
- AT <40% of predicted VO_2max.

As stroke volume is lower in a deconditioned individual, their HR must climb more rapidly to achieve the same cardiac output as someone fitter. Such subjects also have impaired O_2 extraction within muscles. There is, therefore, a shallow profile of the O_2 pulse over time (or steepening of the graph of HR against VO_2).

Deconditioning produces a similar pattern of change in both mild cardiac disease and mild myopathies. These diagnoses may be separated by the subject's complaint of chest pain or marked muscle cramps around the time of the test, or by other tests such as muscle biopsy or myocardial scanning if indicated. A pleasing way to confirm the diagnosis of deconditioning is to retest the individual after a program of exercise and demonstrate an improvement in the O_2 pulse and VO_2max.

15.9 **Obesity**

Most obese subjects are unfit. During a CPEX on a cycle ergometer, they have to do a bit of extra work to move their legs round, but this is less marked than when they are on a treadmill having to move their whole body. This can be seen on a VO_2 vs workload plot, which is displaced upwards in this case. The CPEX will show:

- slightly low or normal VO_2max in ml/min
- low VO_2max in ml kg/min
- low HR reserve
- high VE reserve
- AT at 40–50% of predicted VO_2max.

In addition, SpO_2 at rest may be low and will improve during the CPEX.

15.10 **Trained athletes**

It is usually apparent if the subject is a trained athlete (if only from the gear they wear when they turn up for the CPEX). They should show:

- VO_2max >predicted
- low resting HR
- low HR reserve
- low VE reserve
- clear RCP
- maximum O_2 pulse >20 ml/beat
- AT at >60% predicted VO_2max.

When an athlete notices a decline in performance, they often worry that they have some illness. This isn't usually the case, but if you don't see most of the things on this list, then it might be an indication to do some more tests.

From time to time, a CPEX is needed in an individual with excellent baseline fitness who has experienced an unexpected decline in their performance. For example someone who can usually run marathons but now struggles to jog 10 miles clearly needs investigating. However, this subject is still likely to exceed the usual normal values on the CPEX output, as these relate to sedentary individuals. This usually makes interpreting these types of tests challenging, though some help can be gained from standard tables equating athletic performances (e.g. times to run one mile) with VO_2.

Trained individuals have increased cardiac stroke volume, more efficient O_2 extraction in the muscles, and a host of other physiological changes when compared to the rest of us. This leads to changes evident on the CPEX such as a lower resting HR, higher peak O_2 pulse, and increased maximal VE. Despite these adaptations, they still show cardiac limitation with ventilatory reserve, as normal subjects do. The patterns of limitation that come with airways disease, pulmonary hypertension, and cardiovascular disease are therefore the same as described in other chapters. There are, however, the following specific problems that should be looked out for in athletes that report an unexplained limitation to their performance.

15.10.1 **Exercise-induced bronchoconstriction**

Elite athletes are more likely to have asthma than matched controls by objective and symptoms measures. Much of this increase in prevalence is explained by exercise-induced bronchospasm: a fall of more than 10% in forced expiratory volume in 1 s (FEV1) in response to less than 30 min of exercise. During vigorous exercise, there is loss of water from the airways as a result of humidifying large volumes of air breathed in through the mouth. This causes epithelial injury and thus plasma exudation as part of the repair process. Whilst this repair is underway, there is impaired ability to counteract the airway dehydration during exercise, so there is an even greater change in the osmolality of the airway surface liquid. This leads to release of mast cell mediators in susceptible individuals and thus bronchospasm. Breathing in cold air often augments this effect. Considering the aetiology, it is clear that bronchospasm and related symptoms of exercise-induced bronchoconstriction may therefore only become apparent when an individual trains more frequently or in a different environment.

As CPEXs are usually undertaken in warm, humid hospitals and for less than 20 min, they aren't sensitive in picking up this problem, and an alternative strategy should be used. Exercise tests with better predictive performance have been designed but require specific equipment and have the potential to cause marked bronchospasm. Most centres now use the alternative strategy of inhaled hyperosmolar aerosols, such as dry powder mannitol, to induce airway dehydration.

15.10.2 **Laryngeal dysfunction**

Exercise-induced laryngeal obstruction is relatively common in young, usually female, athletes with symptoms of disproportionate breathlessness on exercise. There is often a concern over a potential asthma diagnosis. The laryngeal obstruction peaks at maximal exercise, at which time the accompanying stridor will be audible but will cease with reduction in load. Flow-volume loops often show inspiratory limitation at peak exercise, which may well persist more subtly into recovery. A definitive diagnosis, however, can only be made by laryngoscopy during exercise, and this is sometimes necessary in specialist centres testing elite athletes. The airflow obstruction and ventilatory changes tend not to significantly impair VO_2max.

Practical tip
Look at the flow-volume plot if the subject's breathing gets noisy during a CPEX.

15.10.3 **Hypertrophic cardiomyopathy**

Trained individuals have some increase in left ventricular wall thickness, and occasionally there is a need to differentiate this process from early hypertrophic cardiomyopathy

(HCM) when a subject has unexplained limitation or symptoms. Large case series of individuals with HCM show that more than a third develop significant outflow-tract gradients on exercise that are not present at rest nor demonstrated upon performing the Valsalva manoeuvre. Hence, distinguishing the trained normal heart from the abnormal can be less straightforward for the referring physician than simply doing an electrocardiogram (ECG) or an echocardiogram. As almost half of sudden cardiac deaths in younger people are due to HCM, it is sensible to have a low threshold for sending these patients along for CPEX to try to make or refute the diagnosis.

In borderline cases, there may not be the significant drop in cardiac output and blood pressure which would be seen in an established case of HCM. For athletes whose sport involves endurance training, the major difference will be that healthy individuals with a little ventricular increase will have a VO_2max more than 20% greater than predicted, whereas the VO_2max for patients with early HCM will often be in the normal range for sedentary individuals. Difficulty can arise with strength athletes, such as weightlifters, as they do not have a supranormal VO_2max. In these cases, however, there may be clues from the early rise in HR in HCM compensating for the reduced maximal stroke volume (early plateau in O_2 pulse) from impaired ventricular relaxation.

Further reading

Anderson SD, Silverman M, Tai E, Godfrey S. Specificity of exercise in exercise-induced asthma. Br Med J. 1971 Dec 25;4(5790):814–15. PubMed PMID: 5135258. Pubmed Central PMCID: 1799719.

Eliasson AH, Phillips YY, Rajagopal KR, Howard RS. Sensitivity and specificity of bronchial provocation testing. An evaluation of four techniques in exercise-induced bronchospasm. Chest. 1992 Aug;102(2):347–55. PubMed PMID: 1643912.

Mancini DM, Eisen H, Kussmaul W, Mull R, Edmunds LH, Jr, Wilson JR. Value of peak exercise oxygen consumption for optimal timing of cardiac transplantation in ambulatory patients with heart failure. Circulation. 1991 Mar;83(3):778–86. PubMed PMID: 1999029.

Sorajja P, Allison T, Hayes C, Nishimura RA, Lam CS, Ommen SR. Prognostic utility of metabolic exercise testing in minimally symptomatic patients with obstructive hypertrophic cardiomyopathy. Am J Cardiol. 2012 May 15;109(10):1494–8. PubMed PMID: 22356797.

Taivassalo T, Jensen TD, Kennaway N, DiMauro S, Vissing J, Haller RG. The spectrum of exercise tolerance in mitochondrial myopathies: a study of 40 patients. Brain. 2003 Feb;126(Pt 2):413–23. PubMed PMID: 12538407.

Chapter 16

Preoperative cardiopulmonary exercise testing

Key points

- Preoperative cardiopulmonary exercise testing is useful in assessing operative risk.
- Maximum oxygen uptake (VO_2max) is the most important parameter.
- The lower the VO_2max, the higher the risk of surgery.

Several guidelines now advocate the use of a cardiopulmonary exercise test (CPEX) prior to major surgery if there is any doubt about how fit the patient is to proceed.

16.1 VO_2max

Whilst there is no doubt that there is a clear relationship between VO_2max and operative mortality, using a fixed cut-off for VO_2max (e.g. 50% predicted), determined a priori and without reference to the specific intervention that the patient is to undergo, does not seem to be particularly helpful. Also, using historical published data on VO_2max will be of limited relevance to the outcome of an operation using the most modern surgical and anaesthetic techniques.

Learning point

A low preoperative VO_2max is associated with increased risk of post-op complications and death. The lower the VO_2max, the higher the risk.

As VO_2max is expressed in ml kg/min, patients who are obese or have a lot of peripheral oedema will have a falsely low value; if we were to use their lean body mass to calculate VO_2max, the value would be much higher. However, since both obesity and heart failure are associated with higher operative mortality, independent of exercise capacity, it perhaps isn't a bad thing that VO_2max exaggerates their risks. The same caveats apply about using a fixed value as a cut-off to decide whether or not a patient is fit for surgery. Having said that, those involved in making the decision about whether to proceed with surgery may need some guidance as to what the CPEX means. Probably

Table 16.1 Measured and predicted values for oxygen uptake at peak exercise (VO_2max) in an individual undergoing a cardiopulmonary exercise test (CPEX).	
VO_2max as an indicator of disease severity	VO_2max (ml kg/min)
Normal	>20
Mild	16–20
Moderate	10–15
Severe	<10

the best guide is the table which was used previously to assess severity in Chapter 3 (see Table 16.1).

> **Learning point**
>
> *From the physiological viewpoint, a subject with a VO_2max >80% predicted or >20 ml kg/min can probably be considered as low risk for surgery.*

CPEX generally outperforms other prognostic measures, but it makes sense to use the results in conjunction with all the other information when deciding whether or not the risk of an operation is justified.

> **Practical tip**
>
> *Preoperative VO_2max should be used together with other clinical information to assess surgical risk. There are no fixed cut-offs, but the lower the VO_2max, the higher the risk of surgery. It is not possible to use a CPEX to give an exact figure for the risk of surgery.*

16.2 **Anaerobic threshold and operative risk**

There is quite a lot of interest in the use of anaerobic threshold (AT) to determine the risk of surgery. The thinking goes that anaerobic metabolism is pretty inefficient, so assessing aerobic capacity should be better than assessing VO_2max, which includes both aerobic and anaerobic processes.

Secondly, VO_2max is dependent on how hard the subject tries. If they quit a bit early, VO_2max will be lower than it could have been, but the AT will be unaffected—provided they have passed the AT and provided it can be determined reliably, which is not always the case.

However, in practice, not everyone has a clear AT. Also, there can be quite a large discrepancy between the various methods for determining the AT. For these reasons, AT isn't as good as VO_2max for determining operative risk.

> **Practical tip**
>
> *VO_2max is a better predictor of operative risk than AT.*

16.3 Work efficiency

Work efficiency is a measure of the aerobic metabolic cost of performing external work, i.e. VO_2/W. This ratio is remarkably constant during exercise in normal subjects, at approximately 10 ml min^{-1} W^{-1} (Figure 16.1). It is therefore an appealing measure to assess fitness, as it does not appear to rely on the subject exercising maximally or the assessor looking up sets of reference ranges by sex, age, or height.

However, the linearity of this slope is fortuitous rather than the result of a constant cost of work, so the relationship can be perturbed by technical factors. For example, repeated testing in the same individual using different ramp rates or pedalling cadence will give differing results. This is a relevant practical issue, as the slope can't be mathematically derived from steady state sub-maximal exercise tests in those with significant heart or lung disease.

More significantly, work efficiency gives little, if any, clue as to the aetiology of exercise limitation and also is poor at picking up mild impairment: VO_2/W goes down with training because less oxygen (O_2) needs to be transported to the muscles, but it also goes down with disease, as less O_2 *can* be transported to the exercising muscles.

16.4 Other parameters

In patients with heart failure, ventilatory slope outperforms VO_2max when assessing operative risk; but it is unclear if this is a consequence of the 'standardization' of VO_2max by weight. Some recent studies have got a bit carried away with derived indices, in an attempt to improve the prognostic value of a CPEX. The reproducibility of these indices and the small size of the studies make it difficult to come up with any useful recommendations at this stage.

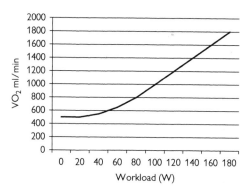

Fig. 16.1 Workload and oxygen uptake (VO_2).

Further reading

Dharancy S, Lemyze M, Boleslawski E, Neviere R, Declerck N, Canva V, et al. Impact of impaired aerobic capacity on liver transplant candidates. Transplantation. 2008 Oct 27;86(8):1077–83. PubMed PMID: 18946345.

Forshaw MJ, Strauss DC, Davies AR, Wilson D, Lams B, Pearce A, et al. Is cardiopulmonary exercise testing a useful test before esophagectomy? Ann Thorac Surg. 2008 Jan;85(1):294–9. PubMed PMID: 18154826.

Hightower CE, Riedel BJ, Feig BW, Morris GS, Ensor JE, Jr, Woodruff VD, et al. A pilot study evaluating predictors of postoperative outcomes after major abdominal surgery: Physiological capacity compared with the ASA physical status classification system. Br J Anaesth. 2010 Apr;104(4):465–71. PubMed PMID: 20190255.

Richter Larsen K, Svendsen UG, Milman N, Brenoe J, Petersen BN. Exercise testing in the preoperative evaluation of patients with bronchogenic carcinoma. Eur Respir J. 1997 Jul;10(7):1559–65. PubMed PMID: 9230247.

Smetana GW. Preoperative pulmonary evaluation. N Engl J Med. 1999 Mar 25;340(12):937–44. PubMed PMID: 10089188.

Snowden CP, Prentis JM, Anderson HL, Roberts DR, Randles D, Renton M, et al. Submaximal cardiopulmonary exercise testing predicts complications and hospital length of stay in patients undergoing major elective surgery. Ann Surg. 2010 Mar;251(3):535–41. PubMed PMID: 20134313.

Bibliography

Reference Texts

American College of Sports Medicine. ACSM's Guidelines for Exercise Testing and Prescription, 8th revised edition (2009) Lippincott Williams and Wilkins.

American College of Sports Medicine. ACSM's Resource Manual for Guidelines for Exercise Testing and Prescription, 8th edition (2009) Lippincott Williams and Wilkins.

Cooper CB, and Storer TW. Exercise Testing and Interpretation: A Practical Approach (2001) Cambridge University Press.

Froelicher VF, Myers JN. Manual of Exercise Testing, 3rd edition (2006) Mosby.

Palange P, Ward S. Clinical Exercise Testing. European Respiratory Monograph (volume 12 monograph 40) (2007) European Respiratroy Society Journals Ltd.

Wasserman K, Hansen JE, Sue DY, Stringer WW, and Whipp BJ. Principles of Exercise Testing and Interpretation: Including Pathophysiology and Clinical Applications, 4th edition (2004) Lippincott Williams and Wilkins.

Statements from Learned Institutions

American Thoracic Society/American College of Chest Physicians. Statement on cardiopulmonary exercise testing. American Journal of Respiratory and Critical Care Medicine. 2003 167(2): 211–77.

Balady GJ, Arena R, Sietsema K, Myers J, Coke L, Fletcher GF, Forman D, Franklin B, Guazzi M, Gulati M, Keteyian SJ, Lavie CJ, Macko R, Mancini D, Milani RV. Clinician's Guide to cardiopulmonary exercise testing in adults: a scientific statement from the American Heart Association. Circulation. 2010 122(2):191–225.

ERS Task Force (Palange P, Ward SA, Carlsen K-H, Casaburi R, Gallagher CG, Gosselink R, O'Donnell DE, Puente-Maestu L, Schols AM, Singh S and Whipp BJ). Recommendations on the use of exercise testing in clinical practice. European Respiratory Journal. 2007 29: 185–209.

List of learning points

- Most cardiopulmonary exercise test (CPEX) results you look at will be breath-by-breath plots of a symptom-limited maximum test, during which the workload was steadily increased until the subject could no longer keep turning the cycle ergometer.
- A maximum oxygen uptake (VO_2max) greater than 80% predicted means that it is very unlikely that the subject has clinically significant pathology affecting their heart or lungs.
- A VO_2max of less than 20 ml kg/min is low; less than 15 ml kg/min indicates moderate impairment of cardiorespiratory function; and less than 10 ml kg/min indicates severe impairment.
- The expected normal value for VO_2max is less in females than in males and declines with age.
- At peak exercise, a normal subject **should** reach 80% or more of their predicted maximum HR.
- Oxygen (O_2) pulse can be used as an indirect indicator of cardiac stroke volume.
- A normal subject should achieve an O_2 pulse of at least 10 ml/beat during a CPEX.
- If the O_2 pulse reaches a plateau, suspect impairment of cardiac output (due to heart disease or pulmonary vascular disease), particularly if the peak value is less than 10 ml/beat.
- Ventilation should **not** reach 80% of predicted during a CPEX in a normal subject.
- If VO_2max is low and ventilation exceeds 80% of predicted (i.e. there is a low ventilatory reserve), then there is probably something wrong with the lungs.
- During a CPEX, carbon dioxide (CO_2) comes from burning O_2 as fuel (aerobic metabolism) and from buffering hydrogen ions (H^+) from lactic acid (generated by anaerobic metabolism).
- The respiratory exchange ratio (RER; carbon dioxide output (VCO_2)/oxygen uptake (VO_2)) should be less than 1.0 in the early part of a CPEX.
- Aerobic metabolism continues beyond the aerobic threshold (AT) but supplemented by anaerobic processes.
- Beyond the AT, VCO_2 increases more steeply than VO_2.
- The AT should be 40% or more of the predicted VO_2max, not the actual VO_2max.
- The presence of a clear respiratory compensation point (RCP) implies the development of sufficient lactic acid to produce acidaemia.

- If the $VEqCO_2$ do not fall below 30, this implies that there is something wrong with gas exchange in the lungs (with a high dead space volume (Vd)/tidal volume (Vt) ratio). Most commonly, this is pulmonary vascular disease.
- A fall in peripheral oxygen saturation (SpO_2) of >4% during a CPEX is abnormal and implies the presence of lung disease, pulmonary vascular disease, or the opening of a right-to-left shunt.
- A CPEX is an excellent way of stressing the gas exchange capabilities of the lungs and unmasking diffusion limitation which may not have been apparent on tests done with the patient at rest.
- Atrial septal defects are common and may only open up on exercise.
- A low preoperative VO_2max is associated with increased risk of post-op complications and death. The lower the VO_2max, the higher the risk.
- From the physiological viewpoint, a subject with a VO_2max >80% predicted or >20 ml kg/min can probably be considered as low risk for surgery.

List of practical tips

- A careful clinical assessment and a few simple tests beforehand will make interpretation of a cardiopulmonary exercise test (CPEX) very much easier.
- The workload-vs-time plot will indicate the different phases of CPEX graphs when they are presented in an unfamiliar format.
- Always check the numbers on the Y-axis of a CPEX plot: some computerized systems will 'autoscale' the graph to fill the whole plot.
- Supervising a CPEX is more informative than simply reviewing the printed results.
- Ventricular ectopics which are present on the resting electrocardiogram (ECG) often disappear on exercise. If they start to occur in runs, stop the CPEX.
- Falling peripheral oxygen saturation (SpO_2) during exercise suggests significant pathology. However, saturations detected by finger probe can fall if the subject grips the handlebars tightly. If you see desaturation during exercise, ask the patient to relax their grip on the bars and think about switching to an earlobe sensor. If the SpO_2 jumps up quickly, then the desaturation was an artefact: real falls in SpO_2 recovery slowly when the subject stops exercising.

- Don't stop a CPEX just because the subject has reached their predicted heart rate (HR): keep going until they have to stop because of symptoms (unless, of course, they develop dysrhythmias, etc).
- 'Did the subject fail to reach 80% or more of their predicted HR?' and 'Was there an abnormally high HR reserve?' are the same question.
- There are quite a few things that influence the oxygen (O_2) pulse. Beware of over-interpreting a low peak O_2 pulse (or a plateau), particularly if the maximum oxygen uptake (VO_2max) is normal.
- Trained athletes can push themselves well beyond the predicted VO_2max. Their stroke volume is such that they can increase their cardiac output considerably, so they continue to exercise for longer and stray into the region where they reach predicted ventilation. This does not imply that there is anything wrong with their lungs.
- An erratic respiratory exchange ratio (RER) during a CPEX is a pointer to the diagnosis of dysfunctional breathing.
- Always look at the graphical display to check which point has been chosen to be called the anaerobic threshold (AT).
- If there is a clear respiratory compensation point (RCP), significant lung disease is unlikely.

- Look for irregularity in minute ventilation (VE), RER, and ventilatory equivalents for carbon dioxide (VEqCO$_2$) in order to distinguish dysfunctional breathing from lung disease.

- When learning to look at an ECG, leads are looked at in a fairly systematic order: I, II, III, aVR, aVL, aVF, and then the V leads. A similar approach should be adopted when starting to look at CPEX graphs, looking first along Graphs 1, 2, and 3 from left to right on the top row, then on to 4, 5, and 6 from left to right on the middle row, and finishing off with 7, 8, and 9 on the bottom row.

- Don't over-interpret the graphs of a CPEX if the VO$_2$max is normal: significant pathology is unlikely.

- CPEX results are presented in lots of different ways. Looking through the data and graphs systematically allows the brain to learn where to find the information that it wants. At first, it may help to use a highlighter pen on a paper copy of the results, circling key points on the graphs or tables and drawing lines between them.

- Look at the flow-volume plot if the subject's breathing gets noisy during a CPEX.

- Preoperative VO$_2$max should be used with other clinical information to assess surgical risk. There are no fixed cut-offs, but the lower the VO$_2$max, the higher the risk of surgery. It is not possible to use a CPEX to give an exact figure for the risk of surgery.

- The VO$_2$max is a better predictor of operative risk than the AT.

Index